"In *Goodnight Mind*, Colleen Carney and Rachel Manber have taken the complex processes needed to establish consistently good sleep and laid out a straightforward set of easy-to-follow guidelines. Nothing is left out of this book—from understanding your body's sleep clock to relaxation and quieting your mind. Carney and Manber have drawn on their years of clinical research experience to develop a rich and accessible resource for those struggling with this tenacious problem."

> —**Donn Posner, PhD, CBSM**, clinical associate professor of psychiatry and human behavior at the Alpert Medical School at Brown University, and coauthor of *The Cognitive Behavioral Treatment of Insomnia*

"We live in a busy, mentally challenging world, and keeping an alert and active mind throughout the day helps us cope with and effectively meet the challenges we face. Unfortunately for the millions of folks with chronic insomnia, persistent thinking, worrying, or more general sleep-disruptive mental arousal serve as the crux of their chronic sleep problems. Fortunately, there are a variety of effective strategies for 'putting the mind to bed' and regaining the ability to sleep normally once again. Those strategies are clearly and comprehensively presented in this new self-help guide by Carney and Manber, two renowned experts in the area of insomnia treatment. This easy-to-read guide provides ten simple steps for keeping one's mind out of the way of a good night's sleep. I am certain that this guide will be a great aid to those who read it."

> —**Jack Edinger, PhD**, professor and director of the behavioral sleep medicine program at National Jewish Health

goodnight mind

turn off your noisy
thoughts & get a
good night's sleep

colleen e. carney, phd
rachel manber, phd

Publisher's Note

This publication is designed to provide accurate and authoritative information in regard to the subject matter covered. It is sold with the understanding that the publisher is not engaged in rendering psychological, financial, legal, or other professional services. If expert assistance or counseling is needed, the services of a competent professional should be sought.

Distributed in Canada by Raincoast Books

Copyright © 2013 by Colleen E. Carney and Rachel Manber
New Harbinger Publications, Inc.
5674 Shattuck Avenue
Oakland, CA 94609
www.newharbinger.com

Cover design by Amy Shoup; Acquired by Jess O'Brien; Edited by Will DeRooy

Library of Congress Cataloging-in-Publication Data

Carney, Colleen.
 Goodnight mind : turn off your noisy thoughts and get a good night's sleep /
Colleen E. Carney, PhD, and Rachel Manber, PhD.
    pages cm
 Includes bibliographical references.
 ISBN 978-1-60882-618-6 (pbk. : alk. paper) -- ISBN 978-1-60882-619-3 (pdf
e-book) -- ISBN 978-1-60882-620-9 (epub) 1. Insomnia--Treatment. 2.
Affective disorders--Treatment. 3. Cognitive therapy. I. Manber, Rachel. II.
Title.
 RC548.C364 2013
 616.8'4982--dc23

                                       2013006046

Printed in the United States of America

15   14   13
10   9   8   7   6   5   4   3   2   1
First printing

Contents

Introduction

Given that you are reading this book, you may have difficulty sleeping or you may have difficulty shutting off your mind when you want to sleep. This is a very common problem, and luckily there are simple strategies to help. The most effective way to address these problems is with tools from cognitive behavioral therapy, or CBT. CBT is an approach to psychology that developed out of research into what causes sleep problems and fatigue. Knowing what causes these problems helped psychologists like us develop solutions to them. CBT is a very well tested, effective treatment approach with many tools that can be used to help you with your sleep problems.

What Causes Sleep Problems?

Many factors influence sleep. In particular, your behaviors, the way you think about sleep, and other factors exert a strong influence on how well you sleep. No matter what initially *caused* your sleep problems—stress, medication, or something else—the way you think or behave can have a negative effect on your sleep and become the primary factor in *sustaining* your sleep problems. If you understand this basic fact, you can make changes in your thinking, your habits, or your environment that will have a positive impact on your sleep. CBT has discovered the type of thinking and the type of habits that foster good sleep, and this book will teach you how to implement these CBT strategies.

Who Should Use This Book?

If your sleep problems have led to trouble during the day, such as difficulty with everyday activities, or if they cause you distress, you may have already been diagnosed with insomnia. Perhaps you have chronic insomnia—for at least a month now, it has taken you over thirty minutes to fall asleep most nights. Yet you need not have any diagnosis in order to benefit from the strategies in this book. If you simply have difficulty falling asleep or staying asleep, or you do not feel *rested* when you wake up, this book can help.

You may wonder whether this book will be helpful if you also have another condition, such as chronic pain, depression, or another medical problem. The good news is that CBT for insomnia is often effective even when there is another condition present.

Being more of a "morning person" or a "night owl" does not necessarily mean you have sleep problems. Many people have some degree of morning or evening tendency. But if the time at which you fall asleep varies from night to night (that is, sometimes you can fall asleep earlier and sometimes you can't fall asleep until much later) even though you are trying to keep a regular schedule, this is suggestive of insomnia, and you can benefit from using the strategies in this book.

Who Might Not Benefit

Those with sleep problems other than insomnia may not benefit from this book. If you doze off unintentionally during the day or evening, tell your doctor, as this can be a sign of another sleep disorder, such as sleep apnea syndrome or periodic limb movement disorder. An overnight study in a sleep laboratory is often needed to rule out these conditions.

If you have difficulty either falling asleep or waking up *at a conventional time*—meaning you are an extreme morning person or night owl—but still get seven to nine hours of sleep, this may be a sign of another disorder called a circadian rhythm disorder. Someone who does not feel sleepy until four in the morning and wakes up feeling refreshed at noon may have this type of disorder. So may someone who falls asleep around eight in the evening and wakes up ready to start the day at four in the morning. In other words, if you consistently go to bed and rise very early or very late but you do not have trouble falling asleep or staying asleep, consult with a sleep specialist to see whether you have a circadian rhythm disorder rather than insomnia.

This book is also not appropriate for those whose sleep problems are due to the fact that they work nights or rotating shifts. Shift work can create tremendous sleep and quality-of-life problems beyond the scope of insomnia, and an entire book would be necessary to deal with the complexities of those issues. If you are having sleep problems relating to shift work, seek professional help from a sleep center.

What to Expect in This Book

A noisy mind interferes with sleep. This book breaks down the problem of a noisy mind into ten steps, ten individual strategies that will help you quiet the mind and improve your sleep. The chapters are meant to be read in order, but some of the chapters may not apply to you, in which case you may focus on particular steps or strategies.

The first chapter will teach you how important it is to understand your sleep system. This chapter provides a simple explanation of how you can get sleep to work for you, rather than you working to get sleep. After reading this chapter, you will understand that a quiet mind is more likely if you *set the stage* for quality sleep. The next two chapters (2 and 3) provide direct instructions on how to start keeping a good sleep schedule and how to build a strong drive for deep, satisfying sleep. Chapter 4 will teach you how to train your active mind to be quiet in bed and how to search through your sleep environment to find any culprits that could be causing an overactive mind. Chapter 5 teaches you how to implement a Buffer Zone, or a time in which your mind can deal with the day's events without getting in the way of sleep. Chapter 6 addresses a noisy mind that stems from tension and anxiety, by teaching you how to start a relaxation practice. Chapter 7 focuses specifically on proven techniques to manage mental overactivity characterized by worry. Chapter 8 will teach you to adopt the mental habits of a good sleeper. Chapter 9 will focus on how to think about and manage fatigue so that it doesn't lead to a noisy mind or sleeplessness at night. Chapter 10 deals with the important role of acceptance in managing unwanted thoughts on troubled nights.

We hope that you enjoy the book, start working through the steps, and start getting the sleep of your dreams!

Chapter 1

Know the Recipe for Good Sleep

There are three key ingredients to getting a good night's sleep. You may believe that all you need to do in order to sleep better is "quiet your mind"; however, your current sleep habits may be making it hard for you to sleep well on a regular basis, or you may be doing certain other things that get in the way of a good night's sleep. These things are easy to change, and if you adjust your sleep system, your noisy mind may resolve itself.

In order to know whether you need to make an adjustment, it is helpful to know the recipe for good sleep and to understand the basic workings of your body's sleep system. This chapter provides a simple explanation of how sleep is produced and an introduction to the idea of how you can get sleep to work for you, rather than you working to get sleep. A quiet mind is more likely if you "set the stage" for quality sleep and have realistic expectations for normal sleep.

Stop Trying to Sleep Well

Ask any good sleeper, "What's your recipe for good sleep?" and you are likely to receive a puzzled look. Or perhaps he or she will say something like, "I don't do anything. I get into bed, and eventually I fall asleep." Ask a dozen *poor* sleepers about their recipe for sleep, however, and you will probably get a dozen different replies:

- "I use a white noise machine and a blackout mask."

- "I drink a glass of wine."

- "I go to bed early and watch television."

- "If I'm not asleep within an hour, I take a sleeping pill."

- "I drink a special tea that is supposed to make me sleepy."

- "If I've had a bad night, I sleep in to try to catch up on lost sleep."

- "I take a sleeping pill on most nights, but after a few bad nights I take a different type of sleeping pill."

- "I listen to the sounds of whale calls and sleep in a separate room from my husband."

- "I listen to a self-hypnosis CD."

- "I sleep in on weekends to try to catch up on lost sleep."

- "I exercise right before bed."

- "I drink warm milk."

- "I take a melatonin supplement."

What do all of these strategies have in common? *Effort*. Those with sleep problems exert tremendous effort to set the stage for sleep, but this is unfortunately the opposite of what needs to occur for sleep. Your body has a built-in system that makes up for poor sleep, and you need not use any effort at all to sleep or make up for lost sleep. In fact, such efforts only interfere with this system and make it more likely that you will have continued sleep problems. Moreover, you may believe that your only problem is that your brain will not "shut down" at night; however, you may be unaware that the problem is rather with your sleep system, and your overactive mind occurs simply because you are already awake in bed. We will provide a recipe for good sleep so that you can identify anything that may be causing your problems. If you find that you have some of the problems described in this chapter, chapters 2 and 3 will provide more detailed, step-by-step solutions.

Know How Your Sleep System Works

There are two main systems that work together to produce sleep: the body clock and the sleep driver.

The Body Clock

The body clock, also called the circadian system, controls when you feel sleepy and when you feel alert. The body clock is actually a system of clocks throughout your body, coordinated by a clock in your brain. If you are like most adults, during the day the body clock produces chemical signals that make you feel alert, and by the evening, the signals fade away. This means there is a nighttime window in which it is optimal for you to sleep, and this "sleep window" remains somewhat fixed unless something changes the system. Events that could change the system include traveling across time zones or a change in the timing of your exposure to sunlight. Have you ever crossed multiple time zones in a single day? If you have, what did you notice the next day with regard to when you became hungry? When you became sleepy? The effect of the sunlight (or lack of sunlight)? In chapter 3, you can take a test to determine your sleep window and learn how to make the body clock work best for you, but for now, it is important to note that our first key ingredient for good sleep is:

1. A regular and optimally timed sleep opportunity (sleep window)

The Sleep Driver System

Sleep is also controlled by a sleep driver system, called the homeostatic system. The sleep driver system balances sleep and wakefulness. It builds a drive for deep sleep from the moment you are awake and out of bed. The longer you are awake and the more active you are, the greater the drive for deep, continuous sleep the next night. When you are sleep deprived, the drive becomes increasingly intense, but alerting signals from the body clock can still enable you to function during the day. Nonetheless, when given the chance to sleep after you have been building sleep drive, you sleep more deeply. This is the built-in process that makes up for poor sleep—note that, in response to lost sleep, your body produces not necessarily *more* sleep but *deeper* sleep. Deeper sleep helps you feel more rested after periods of sleep deprivation. Being physically inactive or spending a lot of time in bed keeps sleep drive from building. The result of decreased sleep drive may be that it takes you longer to fall asleep, or your sleep may be lighter and you may be more vulnerable to frequent waking.

Aim for Quality, not Quantity

It is time to look at quantity versus quality of sleep. Which of the following would you prefer?

A. Six hours of high-quality sleep

B. Eight hours of poor sleep

If your answer is "B," chapter 8 ("Think like a Good Sleeper") may be particularly helpful to you. In Western society, sleep quantity is overvalued, relative to sleep quality. You may believe that you need eight hours to function adequately, but the truth is that there is great variability in the amount of sleep on which you can function.

The media has pushed a message that getting inadequate amounts of sleep can be deadly. For people with sleep problems, this message creates anxiety, but the real picture is not as bleak as you might think. First, it is important to note that studies showing harmful effects of restricting your sleep opportunity have rarely studied people with insomnia only; these studies do not distinguish among the many types of sleep disorders, and neither do they distinguish those who restrict their sleep opportunity voluntarily. For example, some people intentionally spend less time in bed and restrict their sleep opportunity in order to accomplish more during the day or to work multiple jobs. Intentionally restricting your sleep, or having a sleep condition that restricts your sleep, *does* pose health risks.

However, most people with insomnia do not restrict their sleep opportunity. People with insomnia tend to do the opposite; that is, they spend far longer in bed than they are able to sleep. Moreover, people with insomnia often sleep for a normal length of time (on average, they tend to produce six hours or more of sleep), even though it may take them longer to fall asleep or they may be awake for longer during the night.

A good rule of thumb is that you should be sleeping for about 85 percent of the time that you are in bed. You can use a sleep diary (see below) to help you figure out your average percentage. If you are sleeping for more than 90–95 percent of the time that you are in bed, you may be sleep deprived and may need to allow for more time in bed each night. If you are sleeping for less than 80 percent of the time that you are in bed, you may be spending too much time in bed. Chapter 2 will help you determine whether too much time in bed is a problem for you and, if so, will guide you in fixing the problem.

You probably can remember times when you slept for very few hours and actually felt rested, and you probably can also call to mind times when you slept for longer than usual and felt groggy. To improve the quality of your sleep is a better goal than to increase the amount of sleep you get. We will talk more about setting your expectations in a sleep-promoting, rather than sleep-interfering, way in chapters 8 and 9.

Keep a Sleep Diary

Much of the advice we will offer to help you improve your sleep relies on you to systematically track your sleep, because people tend to underestimate how much sleep they get. As soon as possible, begin keeping a diary about your sleep habits. You can use a chart like the one shown at the end of this chapter (also available for download at www.newharbinger.com/26186), or simply write notes on a separate piece of paper each day. Record the following information about the previous night's sleep. Doing this soon after you wake up can help you remember these details more accurately.

1. What time you got into bed (this may not be the time that you began "trying" to fall asleep)

2. About how long it took you to fall asleep

3. The total amount of time you were awake between the time you first fell asleep and your final awakening

4. The time of your final awakening, in other words, the very last time you woke up for the day.

5. What time you got out of bed for the day

Try the following experiment. Keep a sleep diary, and after a week determine the total time you spent in bed. Divide this total time by 7 to find how much time you spent in bed each night on average. Now add up all the time you spent awake, including at the beginning of each night (number 2), in the middle of each night (number 3), and in the morning hours (the difference between number 4 and number 5) and then subtract it from the total time you spent in bed. Divide the result by 7 to find how much sleep you got on average each night. If you want, you can divide this by the time you spent in bed each night on average and then multiply the result by 100 to come up with a percentage.

You may assume that you are sleep deprived and so you must be building good sleep drive; however, take a look at your time spent in bed and compare it to how much time you spent asleep. Is there a big difference? Is your average amount of time spent in bed eight hours or more? Let's say you can only produce, on average, five and a half hours of sleep—if you spent eight hours in bed (i.e., you were asleep only about 69 percent of the time you were in bed), this would interfere with building enough sleep drive to produce deep sleep the next night. Moreover, you might try to make up for how badly you felt the next day by canceling plans (i.e., becoming less active), cutting back on exercise, attempting to nap, sleeping in, or going to bed earlier than usual. All of these prevent a strong drive for deep sleep. If any of this sounds like you, or if you are yearning for a higher quality of sleep, be sure to read chapter 2. For now, it is important to remember our second ingredient for good sleep:

2. A strong drive for sleep

Your Arousal or Activation System

The body clock and the sleep driver work together to produce quality sleep, and knowing how to work with these two systems can produce satisfying sleep; however, there is one thing that can trump these two systems and cause sleep problems: the arousal system. The arousal system, which is responsible for making you feel extra alert when necessary, is ideally less active during sleep. It is important that the arousal system be able to override sleep in emergencies—cases of danger (e.g., if your house was being burgled)—so that you can wake up and take appropriate action (e.g., call the police). However, an overactive arousal system interferes with sleep, especially because the system is not very good at determining which dangers are true and immediate ones that require wakefulness. For example, if we tell participants in a research experiment that in the morning, they will have to give a public speech, we can expect that their sleep will be worse than if we had not created this anxiety. The supposed public speech is not until the morning, so the danger of embarrassment is not immediate, but the anticipation of something stressful can create arousal and interfere with sleep.

Spot (and Address) Things That Interfere with Sleep

Arousal is a state of emotional, physical, or mental activation incompatible with sleep. Look over the following list. Which things do you think can produce significant arousal and interfere with sleep? Which, on the other hand, are relaxing and promote better sleep?

Alcohol	Staying in bed while awake	A cold bedroom
Thinking about sleep	Cigarettes	Talking on the phone in bed
Reading in bed	Making a to-do list	Anxiety
Stress	A hot bedroom	Pets in your bed
Marijuana	Cold medications	Exercise before bed

You may be surprised to learn that all of these things can be activating and interfere with sleep.

Also, while it is well known that caffeine (such as in chocolate, teas, coffee, and sodas) before bedtime can interfere with quality sleep, most people do not know that even afternoon caffeine can negatively affect sleep. It can be difficult to gauge how much caffeine you are consuming and how efficient your body is at eliminating caffeine from your system before bedtime; people vary. And even substances you may think are calming can be culprits in arousal. For example, many people believe that cigarettes are calming, because many people experience an alleviation of tension once they light up. This tension reduction, however, is actually nothing more than the abating of the nicotine withdrawal symptoms that have been building since the previous cigarette. Cigarettes are actually activating, and the nicotine withdrawal produces agitation. This may be one of the mechanisms behind the addiction to cigarettes; that is, the belief that you need a cigarette to relax, when the cigarette habit may actually cause the tension.

Similarly, many people believe that marijuana and alcohol are sleep-promoting substances, because sometimes they can decrease the time it takes to fall asleep. However, the net result of these substances is poor sleep. Both of these substances suppress rapid eye movement (REM) sleep in the first part of the night, and when the active ingredients in these substances are broken down and metabolized during the night, more REM sleep is produced. REM sleep is not a deep stage of sleep. In fact, it used to be called paradoxical sleep because brain activity during this stage of sleep closely resembles brain activity while awake. During REM sleep, your sleep is lighter, and you are more prone to waking, sweating, and having intense dreams.

There are many medications that can cause sleep problems or make them worse. For example, some cold and allergy medications, particularly those with a decongestant, can cause insomnia. Some asthma or heart medications (e.g., beta blockers) can cause insomnia. When starting any new medication, read the medication insert to find whether insomnia is listed as a possible side effect. Talk to your doctor about whether insomnia could be a side effect of any medications you are currently taking.

One of the items in the above list can, interestingly, be either a sleep-promoter or an arousal-promoter: exercise. Regular exercise improves sleep; however, some exercise routines are activating and energizing and thus should not be done in the evening. We recommend that you engage in regular and even rigorous exercise, but not within two hours of bedtime. Many people try to physically exhaust themselves into falling asleep, only to find themselves even more alert. Exercise that entails stretching and slow movement, such as yoga or tai chi, may promote relaxation and is fine to do as part of a wind-down practice before bed. For more on the importance of a wind-down period, see chapter 5.

The environment in which you sleep can also have an impact on arousal. Extremes in temperature can cause you to wake up throughout the night or can delay the onset of sleep. Some people believe that they need their room to be either hot or cold in order to fall asleep; however, your body goes through many thermoregulatory changes throughout the night, and if your bedroom is too hot or too cold this could be causing you to wake up. It is important that you maintain a comfortable bedroom temperature in order to fall asleep and stay asleep throughout the night. Do you allow pets in your bed? Pets may be a part of your family and a great source of comfort; however, pets can have a negative impact on the depth of your sleep. Pets can snore and make noises throughout the night. Pets can insist that you let them out of the bedroom for a midnight snack. They also shift positions frequently and have little concern for whether you have adequate space for sleeping! If your pet is interfering with your sleep, by waking you up with noises or impinging on a comfortable sleeping posture, it may be time to try something new.

Generally speaking, your bed should be associated with sleep. It should be a space reserved specifically for sleep. When you are in bed, if you engage in activities that you normally do when you are awake—reading, surfing the web, making a to-do list, eating, watching television, talking on the phone, or checking for texts—you are unintentionally training your body to be awake in bed. Anything you do in bed that you might also do when you are your "wakeful self" can ultimately cause and worsen insomnia. Similarly, if you simply spend extended time awake in bed, particularly if you are upset, your bed becomes the place where you are awake, alert, and frustrated. Many years ago, Dr. Ivan Pavlov conducted experiments in which he showed a dog meat and the dog would drool. This is not surprising, as food, particularly meat, naturally causes dogs to drool. Dr. Pavlov did something different next. He rang a bell while showing the dog the meat many times, and each time the dog would drool. After pairing the sound of the bell and the sight of the meat many, many times, he rang the bell without presenting the meat. The result? The dog drooled. Why? The bell had become a signal, or a cue, for drool. Think about the effect on you of pairing your bed night after night with wakefulness and frustration. Your bed loses its power as a signal for sleep and, instead, becomes a signal for wakefulness. This can worsen insomnia. Chapter 4 will provide very specific strategies for un-training your body to be awake at night.

You may find the activities listed above (reading, surfing the web, etc.) relaxing, so the answer may be not to stop these habits, but rather to move them to a different place and time. For more on this topic, read chapter 5.

Now for more obvious arousal-producing culprits: stress, anxiety, and worry. Bedtime can be the first time all day that allows you quiet and undistracted thought, and this unfortunately can lend itself to problem solving, list-making, and planning. These are all good activities for the daytime, but thinking about what will happen tomorrow can set off worry. Chapters 5 through 10 are specifically geared toward helping produce the last ingredient in our sleep recipe:

3. A quiet mind and body, and a comfortable sleep environment

Summary

This chapter introduced you to the workings of your sleep system. Understanding the body clock and the sleep driver system is the first step toward improving your sleep. You now know, for example, that spending too much time in bed can prevent you from getting enough quality sleep, and some things you may have thought were sleep aids can get in the way of a peaceful night's rest. If you can reduce or eliminate activities or substances that produce emotional, physical, or mental activation and can interfere with sleep, you will not need to try so hard to fall asleep. As you read this book, keep in mind our three key ingredients for sleep:

1. A regular and optimally timed sleep opportunity (sleep window)

2. A strong drive for sleep

3. A quiet mind and body, and a comfortable sleep environment

My Sleep Diary

	Monday	Tuesday	Wednesday	Thursday	Friday	Saturday	Sunday
What time you got into bed*							
How long it took you to fall asleep							
The total time you were awake between the time you first fell asleep and your final awakening							
The time of your final awakening							
What time you got out of bed for the day							

* This may not be the time that you began "trying" to fall asleep.

Chapter 2

Build a Stronger Drive for Deep Sleep

As we discussed in chapter 1, one of the main ingredients for good sleep is to build a strong drive for deep sleep. Deep sleep is the type of sleep that gives you longer stretches of continuous or uninterrupted sleep and makes you feel more rested when you wake up. This chapter will teach you how to get your sleep driver system back on track by adjusting your sleep schedule, increasing your activity levels, and adjusting any habits that may be getting in the way of building a strong drive for deep sleep.

Give Your Sleep System a Tune-Up

Have you ever thought about *how* your body produces deep sleep? If you seem to not get enough deep sleep, perhaps you are worried that your body's system for producing deep sleep is broken or has malfunctioned. Luckily, this is rarely the case. In fact, you will be relieved to learn that there are things that you can do to help your sleep system work better for you.

As we mentioned in chapter 1, your body's natural system that balances sleep and wakefulness does not usually make up for lost sleep by producing *more* sleep the following night. It makes up for lost sleep by producing *deeper* sleep. You can get the most of this system merely by understanding how this system works and what behaviors get in the way of the deep sleep you desire. For example, if you spend too little time out of bed, or expend very little energy during the day, the drive may not be strong enough to produce deep, continuous sleep that night. Your drive for deep sleep becomes stronger when you are awake and active for most of the day.

This information can provide some comfort when you are sleeping poorly, because you can count on your body to produce enough deep sleep to make up for lost sleep. This also means that any efforts to make up for lost sleep will backfire; such efforts include going to bed early, staying in bed longer, or attempting to nap. These behaviors may weaken the buildup of a drive for deep sleep. Similarly, to make up for lost sleep you may increase your caffeine consumption, but caffeinated products such as cola and coffee interfere with the buildup of one of the chemicals needed for deep sleep. Efforts to catch up on lost sleep and the use of caffeine are common and understandable responses to sleep loss, but these behaviors send the wrong message to your body and prevent adequate drive for deep sleep.

Strategies for Increasing Deep Sleep

There are several ways you can make your sleep system work for you and get the (deep) sleep of your dreams.

Limit Your Time in Bed

In general, you should spend only about as much time in bed as you can sleep. We will give you detailed guidelines for limiting your time in bed later in this chapter. Even if you choose not to set and observe a new sleep schedule as we recommend, try to follow these two important rules.

Do not sleep in. Spending more time in bed in the morning takes away from how much drive for deep sleep you can build on a given day because, unless you go to bed later the next night, the time for your sleep drive to build is shortened. The sleep you get in the morning hours is not particularly restorative anyway. So, set an alarm and stick to a given rise time (chapter 3 will help you determine the right one for you), and you will be rewarded with a stronger drive for deep sleep.

Do not go to bed early to make up for lost sleep. Going to bed early after a poor night's sleep stops the buildup for deep sleep too early. This means that you are unlikely to get enough deep sleep and you may be more likely to wake up in the middle of the night.

Do Not Nap

Napping during the day robs you of some of the deep sleep you would get at night. When you get up from a nap, you have to rebuild the sleep drive you lost, and it is unlikely that you will have built a strong enough drive for deep sleep by the time you go to bed for the night. When you get less deep sleep, your sleep may seem less restful and you may wake up in the middle of the night.

Avoid Dozing ("Nodding Off")

Nodding off and dozing have the same negative effects as napping and should be avoided. Use an activity—preferably one with physical movement—and bright light to manage the urge to doze. If you can, ask someone to wake you up if they see you dozing. Avoid situations that make it more likely you will doze, such as watching television or movies in low light, or reclining on a couch or chair in the evening.

Be Active during the Day

Increasing your activity levels is good for your health, your mood, and your sleep. Being physically active builds more sleep drive and can increase deep sleep. If you are awake but inactive or resting for most of the day, you are less likely to be able to have a deep, sound sleep.

Limit or Eliminate Caffeine

Since caffeine interferes with the buildup of sleep drive and can reduce sleep quality, limit your intake. Consume no more than 250 milligrams of caffeine per day (a 12-ounce mug of coffee has just over half this amount), and try not to have any caffeine within six hours of your bedtime. If you are particularly sensitive to caffeine, you may need to restrict your caffeine to mornings or eliminate it altogether.

Reduce the Time You Spend in Bed

The strategy above—"Spend only about as much time in bed as you can sleep"—is one of the most effective ways to achieve deeper sleep. Many people are unclear about how to spend only as much time in bed as the amount of sleep they produce, because the amount of sleep they get varies from one night to the next, sometimes greatly. The key to determining how much time you should spend in bed is to figure out how much sleep you get on average. When asked to estimate their average amount of sleep, people tend to remember their worst nights, so without hard data, underestimation is a risk (one that can have consequences for your efforts to improve your sleep). A sleep diary can paint a more accurate picture of your sleep pattern.

Step 1: Record Your Sleep

The best way to discover how much sleep you get on average is to write down a few details about your sleep each morning for two weeks. You can use a sleep diary as described in chapter 1. When you are recording information about your sleep, the sooner in the day you do it, the more accurate it will be, so try to prioritize completing your sleep diary entry early in the morning. You may find that leaving your sleep diary and a pen either on your nightstand or at the breakfast table increases the likelihood that you will fill it out consistently and accurately.

Do this starting now: record information on your sleep for two weeks, and do not read any further in this book until you have. You may be tempted to skip this step and keep reading, but the way to get the best results is to first have accurate information about your sleep. In the meantime, you can use what you have learned so far to set the stage for a better night's sleep. Place a bookmark here for now....

Step 2: Figure Out How Much Time You Spent in Bed

Welcome back! Now, what is the average difference between the time you got into bed and the time at which you got out of bed over the past two weeks? That is, how much time did you spend in bed? For example, if you got into bed at 10:00 p.m. to watch television and then got out of bed at 7:00 a.m., you spent nine hours in bed. Figure out how much time you spent in bed each night and total these times, then divide by the number of days you monitored your sleep (14, if you monitored for two weeks, as we suggest). This will give you your average time spent in bed per night. People who have sleep difficulties are often surprised by how much time they spend in bed each night. Nine hours in bed is not unusual. However, most adults cannot produce nine hours of sleep, so spending this much time in bed makes it more likely that you will be awake in bed and that you will spend less time building sleep drive out of bed.

Step 3: Figure Out How Much Time You Spent Sleeping

To find how much actual sleep you got, subtract the length of time you were awake in bed from the length of time that you were in bed. For example, if you were in bed for nine hours and it took you an hour to fall asleep, you spent ninety minutes awake in the middle of the night, and you did not get out of bed for an hour after you woke up in the morning (maybe you tried to get back to sleep), the time spent awake in bed was three and a half hours, so actual sleep time was five and a half hours. To arrive at the average amount of sleep your body produced, add together the times spent asleep on each of the nights you monitored and then divide the sum by the number of days you monitored your sleep (14, if you monitored for two weeks, as we suggest).

Step 4: Figure Out How Much Time You Should Spend in Bed Each Night

Now that you have calculated the average amount of sleep your body produces, this is essentially the answer to the question of how much time you should spend in bed. To make your sleep driver system work well for you (by producing deeper, more continuous sleep), you should be in bed only for about as long as your body usually sleeps. You can decide to be strict and aim for only the length of time you calculated in step 3, or, if you like, you can add an extra half hour to allow for the fact that even people who sleep well spend some time awake in bed, usually no more than thirty minutes. For example, if your average time spent asleep was five and a half hours, you can spend six hours in bed each night so that you get the amount of sleep you have been getting on average. If the average amount of time you spent asleep was less than four and a half hours, go ahead and give yourself five hours, because if you were to track your sleep for longer than two weeks your average would probably be at least four and a half hours; also, we recommend that you never spend less than five hours in bed, to avoid sleep deprivation. Write down your goal:

I should be spending no more than _____ hours in bed each night.

What is the difference between the time you have been spending in bed on average over the past two weeks and your new time-in-bed recommendation? It is not unusual for there to be more than an hour difference between the two figures. In our example, the difference is at least three hours. The greater the difference, the more your sleep drive will build in the nights to follow.

Step 5: Make and Follow a New Schedule

The number of hours from step 4 is the new length of time you should spend in bed each night, seven nights a week.

If this is six hours, you might set a twelve o'clock bedtime and a six o'clock rise time (see chapter 3 for determining your best rise time). However, do not use your optimal length of time in bed to justify sleeping in if you go to bed late one night; stick to your rise time. That night you will be in bed for a shorter time, but this is okay because it will increase the pressure on the sleep driver to produce more deep sleep the next night.

You should also adhere to your new schedule each night even if you slept poorly the night before. Remember, you are trying to allow your body's system to make up for lost sleep by producing greater amounts of deep sleep. If you give in to the understandable temptation to spend more time in bed in the morning following a night of poor sleep, you will undo the desired effect and will not receive the reward of deep sleep. In fact, you will likely sleep less deeply the following night because you will have spent less time building sleep drive.

If you follow this recommendation consistently, this buildup will eventually translate to deeper sleep. Keep in mind that you are not limiting your sleep by following this recommendation; you are limiting your time spent awake in bed so that you can sleep more efficiently and deeply.

Are You Hesitant to Reduce the Time You Spend in Bed?

You may have mixed feelings about this new sleep habit. Although you may be convinced by the rationale we provided and may even be excited at the prospect of obtaining deeper sleep, you may feel nervous about spending less time in bed. This nervousness usually stems from worrying that if you spend less time in bed you will end up sleeping even less than you have been.

There are a few things to keep in mind. First, decreasing the time you spend in bed is not a recommendation to be followed indefinitely. We recommend that as your sleep improves you slowly spend more time in bed (see the next heading).

Second, you do not know whether you will sleep less. Test it out over the next week or two and then look back and determine whether on average your prediction came true. It is important to follow the recommendation for at least a week to test your prediction, because the amount of sleep you get varies from night to night—this is normal—and it may take a few days before your sleep becomes consistently deeper. In other words, do not worry if you do get less sleep the first few nights—this trend will likely reverse. Give it some time; do not quit before the recommendation has had a chance to work.

Third, if you stick to this reduction of your time in bed, you may notice that you are becoming sleepier as bedtime approaches and may even start having difficulty staying awake. This is a sign that your sleep drive is building. If you take it in stride rather than worry about it, you will soon experience deeper, high-quality sleep. It may take a few days for this to occur, but it will happen. However, if you become very sleepy outside of bed, you must also consider your safety and others'. If you are feeling very sleepy, observe the same cautions as you would if you were taking a sedating medication. That is, avoid driving or operating machinery.

Last, this strategy needs to be followed fairly consistently for it to work. If you are nervous about possibly losing sleep and "play it safe" by spending more time in bed on weekends, your efforts during the workweek will be undone. You will not get the benefits of having spent less time in bed on weeknights—that is, increased deep sleep—because your sleep drive will be weakened by your weekend behavior. Consider this: if you follow a diet during the week but overeat on the weekends, will you lose much weight, if any?

Following a strict schedule is the fastest road to results, but if you still do not feel ready to make such a change, you can take it more slowly and adjust your expectations for how quickly the strategy will work. Remember the basic rules for limiting your time in bed from earlier in this chapter: do not go to bed early, and do not sleep in to try to make up for lost sleep.

Extend the Time You Spend in Bed

Once your sleep has improved significantly and you are feeling very sleepy during the day, you may want to experiment with slowly extending the time you spend in bed. Here are some rules that can guide you in making this determination. A "significant sleep improvement" may be identified in several ways. One way is to ask yourself, *Am I now satisfied with the quality of my sleep?* A second way is to compare your sleep with that of someone who does not have sleep problems. Someone without sleep problems tends to fall asleep within thirty minutes of going to bed and spends less than thirty minutes awake in the middle of the night. This means that for a person without sleep problems, the percentage of time spent asleep is around 85–90 percent of the time spent in bed. If your overall average percentage is 90 percent or greater—that is, you are asleep for almost the entire time that you are in bed—extend your time in bed over the next week by fifteen minutes each night. It is your choice as to whether to set your alarm for fifteen minutes later or go to bed fifteen minutes earlier. Similarly, if it used to take you more than thirty minutes to fall asleep before you began restricting your time in bed, but now you fall asleep much more quickly (say within an average of fifteen minutes or less), give yourself fifteen more minutes.

Importantly, you should also extend your time in bed if you experience considerable sleepiness during the day and are concerned about your safety. This may happen, for example, if you based your new time in bed on an underestimation of how long you sleep, thus limiting your sleep most nights and not just your time in bed. However, do not confuse sleepiness with fatigue. You may be tired but not sleepy; that is, you are not dozing off unintentionally when inactive.

Summary

This chapter went into detail as to how you can build a stronger drive for deep sleep. It emphasized the importance of limiting your time spent in bed. It also highlighted the helpfulness of increasing your activity during the day, eliminating naps and dozing, and being careful with caffeine. Following our guidelines for limiting your time in bed can quickly increase your sleep drive to help you fall asleep within thirty minutes and spend less time awake during the night. Succumbing to the urge to go to bed early or sleep in will reduce the effectiveness of this strategy. Remember the following tips:

- Sometimes your mind is awake because your body is not yet ready for sleep.

- You can create a readiness for deep sleep by limiting the amount of time you spend in bed to match the amount of sleep you can currently produce.

- Any attempt to make up for lost sleep will backfire, because it prevents your body from making up for lost sleep naturally.

Chapter 3

Find and Set a Proper Sleep Schedule

In chapter 1, you learned that if your sleep schedule does not match your body clock, you will not have the quality of sleep you desire. If your mind is too active when you are trying to sleep, the reason could be that you are trying to sleep at a time when your body clock is promoting alertness. This chapter will teach you how to create a set sleep schedule that matches your body clock.

What Is the Body Clock, and Why Is It Important for Sleep?

As we discussed in chapter 1, you have an internal clock that determines the best timing for sleep. Throughout the morning and early part of the day, the body clock sends stronger and stronger alerting, or wakeful, signals; as the day goes on, these signals gradually fade, paving the way for sleepy signals to become dominant. If you go to bed much earlier or much later than your clock expects, you will either have difficulty sleeping or experience poor sleep quality. Because your body clock is so important in determining the quality of your sleep, the time you select for being in bed to sleep must (a) match your body clock type and (b) be regular. Let's start with an exploration of your body clock type and then discuss why regularity leads to better sleep.

Step 1: Pick a Sleep Window That Matches Your Body Clock Type

The first step in finding and setting a sleep schedule is deceptively simple: choose a period for sleeping that matches your body clock type. People have a range of body clock types. At one extreme, there are definite morning types, and at the other end are extreme evening types; everyone else falls somewhere in between. Where are you on this spectrum? If you are unsure of your body clock type, read the descriptions below.

If you have the following tendencies, you are an extreme evening type, also called a night owl:

- You have difficulty waking up in the morning (or others have difficulty waking you up).

- You dislike and avoid eating early in the morning.

- You feel mentally cloudy for a while after waking up in the morning.

- You feel at your best in the evening.

- You become sleepy much later than most others do (for example, later than midnight).

If on the other hand the following are descriptive of you, you are an extreme morning type, also called an early bird, or lark:

- You become sleepy much earlier than most others do (usually earlier than 10:00 p.m.).

- You have difficulty staying awake in the evening.

- You wake up in the morning much earlier than most others do, without an alarm.

- You feel most mentally alert in the morning; this alertness declines throughout the afternoon and into the evening.

Although going to bed early and waking up early—or going to bed late and waking up late—may be in line with your body clock, it may be at odds with your partner's. Your spouse, significant other, friend, family member, or roommate may have trouble understanding that your body clocks are different, so your ideal sleep patterns are different, and efforts to change this may in fact be counterproductive. If you are an extreme night person and your partner is an extreme morning person, it does not mean that your preferred sleep habits are wrong and your partner's are right (or vice versa). Different people simply have different body clocks.

If your new sleep window has the potential to create relationship problems, do your best to communicate with your partner and compromise. Below are some solutions you might explore.

- Explain that your "unusual" sleep window may be biologically based and therefore not easy to change. Because body clocks have a significant genetic component, you may be able to identify at least one person in your family who can sympathize.

- If you are a night person: explain that, for you, waking up at 7:00 a.m. feels just as "off" as waking up at 3:00 a.m. does for most people. Just as most people would find it unappealing to eat breakfast at 3:00 a.m., you do not find it appealing to eat at 7:00 a.m.

- If you are a morning person: explain that, for you, staying in bed trying to sleep later in the morning is just as unpleasant and irritating as it would be for your friend or partner to try to go to sleep at 8:00 p.m.; no doubt your friend or partner would find it difficult to fall asleep so early. Just as most people would feel agitated to have to be in bed for the night when they still had energy, it makes you feel uncomfortable to remain in bed in the morning when your energy is already ramping up.

- Compromise on when you expect each other to do things that require energy. A morning person can reduce demands on a night person in the morning, and a night person can reduce demands on a morning person in the evening. The afternoon may be the best time to enjoy shared activities.

- For couples, accept your differences and agree to go to bed at different times but establish a "tuck-in" or a cuddle period so you can continue spending time together at night. For example, go to bed together and cuddle, but when the morning person is ready to sleep the night person can leave the bedroom and return to bed later when sleepy. Conversely, a night person may appreciate a cuddle in the morning upon waking up. The morning person, who has been up for a while, could return to bed to spend time with the night person. Remember that intimacy can occur independent of a sleep schedule.

Step 2: Maintain Your New Schedule Every Single Day

Once you determine a sleep window (that is, the regular time at which you provide yourself with an opportunity to sleep in bed) that matches your body clock type, you must use this same sleep window night after night. Do not vary your sleep window from one night to the next. Many sleep problems are caused by an irregular schedule, and an irregular schedule can cause insomnia and fatigue.

Are You Suffering from Social Jet Lag?

Jet lag is the result of a mismatch between the local time and the time your body thinks it is, as occurs when you travel significantly east or west by jet. When you are in a different time zone than usual, the clock in your body is no longer in sync with the clock on the wall. Common symptoms of jet lag are insomnia and fatigue. If you experience these symptoms without having traveled, we call this *social jet lag*. Social jet lag occurs when there are societal constraints on your sleep schedule because of work, your children, or other responsibilities such that you cannot keep a schedule consistent with your body clock type. To find out whether you are suffering from social jet lag, keep track of your sleep over the next two weeks (see chapter 1 for detailed instructions on keeping a sleep diary). Every day, as soon as you can after getting out of bed, record what time you physically got into bed and what time you physically got out of bed. These times may be different than when you intended to sleep or what time you woke up; you just need to record the time into and out of bed. For example, if you climbed into bed at nine to read a book for an hour before attempting to go to sleep, and you woke up at five thirty but tried to get another half hour of sleep before your alarm went off at six, just record 9:00 p.m. and 6:00 a.m. for that day. At the end of the two weeks, find the difference between the earliest time you got into bed and the latest time you got into bed.

Then find the difference between the earliest time you got out of bed and the latest time you got out of bed. Is each difference an hour or greater? If so, you can expect symptoms of jet lag the same as if you had crossed a time zone. The greater the difference, the greater the possible changes in sleep, energy levels, and appetite you may have from day to day. For example, if you stay up two hours later than usual on Fridays and Saturdays and sleep in for two hours on Saturdays and Sundays, the effect on your body is much as if you lived in Chicago but traveled to Las Vegas every weekend. Perhaps, then, you can improve your energy and sleep simply by preventing social jet lag.

Pick a Standard Rise Time

For some, picking a standard time to get out of bed is an unappealing idea. Many people do not like getting up in the morning, so the idea of getting up at the same time even on mornings after a poor night's sleep may seem unpleasant. Also, you may wonder, *How do I pick which time I should get up each day?*

There are a few ways to select a standard rise time. First, let's clarify the rules. A rise time is the time at which your feet should be on the floor and you should be out of bed. We say this because many people set an alarm but then do not rise until some time later. The time at which you become active (when you get out of bed for the day and start to go about your business), not the time at which you wake up and hit "snooze," is the time at which you begin building your drive for the following night's sleep.

Here are some questions to help you select the best time to get out of bed.

What is the earliest time at which you routinely have to get out of bed? If you have to be awake at a set time several mornings per week, this set time is often the best place to start.

What time does your body wake up naturally? If your body naturally wakes up much earlier than the regular time at which you get out of bed, it is preferable to rise earlier. For example, if you tend to get out of bed at seven most mornings, but your body wakes you up at five thirty most mornings, this is a clue to your body clock type and you should strongly consider a 5:30 a.m. rise time. If you get out of bed earlier, you will build even more drive for quality sleep by being out of bed for longer during the day; your body is not producing quality sleep anyway when you linger in bed and doze.

If on the other hand your body naturally wakes up much later than your usually scheduled rise time, meaning that you sleep soundly right up until your rise time and have substantial difficulty getting up each morning, you may have difficulty selecting your current earliest rise time as your new set rise time. In that case, if it is generally difficult for you to get out of bed no matter what time you have to get up, here are a few tips:

- Force yourself to get up.

- Expose yourself to bright light.

- Engage in an activity with lots of movement as soon as possible.

This will help you shake off your grogginess so that you can get on with your day more quickly. If you have difficulty getting up because you have a job that requires you to be awake and out of bed much earlier than your body clock would dictate, you can explore ways to save time in the morning so that you can set a slightly later rise time. For example, do whatever you can at night to prepare for the following day (shower, lay your clothes out, set the automatic start on the coffee maker) and remove unnecessary activities from your morning routine. Then stick to this rise time even on your off days, and most likely your body will eventually shift toward being more alert at this earlier time.

"But I Hate Schedules."

Do you have a negative reaction to the idea of keeping a schedule? Why? Is it because you associate routines with childhood? Perhaps when you were growing up, your parents were overly strict or inflexible when it came to routines. Perhaps your mother or father told you things like: "No, you can't watch the fireworks. They start at eight, and that's your bedtime." Maybe you think that following a schedule is too boring or limiting for you—you need freedom to do as you would like and room to be spontaneous.

Keeping regular times for basic human functions such as sleeping and eating does not mean that you cannot be spontaneous. Also, humans do not outgrow the need for routines. Although some people may think that only children need routines to help them regulate their mood and alertness, adults need routines too. Routines help "set" the body clock that regulates sleep, mood, and alertness. Aversion to a schedule may interfere with your ability to make the changes needed for you to sleep better. You may want to consider examining and challenging your beliefs about schedules; it may help remove obstacles to improving your sleep.

After you identify any beliefs about keeping a set rise time that could get in the way of following this recommendation, try this experiment: Set aside your belief that routines are _____ (fill in the negative word or phrase, such as "boring" or "limiting to my freedom") for one month and see how you feel. In other words, commit to following the set schedule for one month (not for life) and see whether avoiding social jet lag leads to an improvement in your sleep and in how you feel during the day.

What about Setting a Regular Bedtime?

If the body clock works best when you keep a regular schedule, then should you set a bedtime? This is a tricky question to answer. It is best to have a set bedtime that matches your body clock; that is, a bedtime that coincides with when you regularly feel sleepy. However, sleepiness also depends on how much sleep drive you have built up over the course of the day, so keeping to a bedtime does not always make sense (a) on nights when you have not yet built enough drive for deep sleep or (b) if you often become upset as bedtime approaches and the resultant distress interferes with your ability to sleep.

The time at which you become sleepy can vary from night to night. However, the time at which you have to get up in the morning is often dependent on external factors such as work or other obligations; therefore, you should focus on establishing a set rise time. By observing this rise time seven days a week, you will begin to feel sleepy around the same time each night. This sense of sleepiness will act as your new cue for bedtime, rather than a precise time on a clock. But remember not to go to bed much earlier than your ideal bedtime (see chapter 2).

If It Does Not Work

If you maintain the exact same rise time every day, this practice should lead to feeling sleepy around the same time every night. However, it should be noted that even with your body clock sending sleepy cues around the same time each night, you may be doing things that interfere with or undermine this natural process. For example, do you remain active and engaged in your environment right up until your bedtime? Do you feel as if you have too much to do at night, preventing you from following a relaxing bedtime routine? Activity can override the sleepy cues or make it difficult for you to actually notice them. A failure to unwind before bedtime will result in an overactive mind and lead to sleep disturbance. For more on the importance of protecting your wind-down period and for help in doing so, see chapter 5.

Summary

This chapter taught you to identify your body clock type to determine your ideal sleep window, the time during which you are most likely to sleep well. You can then set a new sleep schedule. The most important part of your new schedule is your rise time—you should rise at the same time every day. Varying your rise time can lead to social jet lag, which contributes to sleep problems.

You may be reluctant to follow a new sleep schedule, even if it means better sleep for you, if it would conflict with your sleeping partner's schedule. If so, you can avoid friction in the relationship if both of you are understanding and willing to make some adjustments and compromises. If you have objections to scheduling your sleep time because you have a distaste for schedules and routines, experiment with keeping a schedule for a month.

Don't forget:

- Everyone's body clock is different. Accept that your body clock type may not be the same as your partner's or friend's.

- Ensure that your sleep window matches your body clock type.

- Use an alarm to enforce your new rise time.

Chapter 4

Train Your Active Mind to Be Quiet in Bed

Once you have adjusted your sleep habits and you start sleeping better (see chapters 2 and 3), it's time to turn your attention to training your mind to be quiet in bed, so that your time in bed is even more restful. There are many reasons an active mind may keep you awake when you want to be sleeping. This chapter focuses on one common reason: you have unknowingly trained yourself to be alert in bed. In this chapter, you will learn to identify and banish culprits that could be causing this problem. You will also learn how getting out of bed when your mind is noisy will train your mind to be quiet in bed.

How the Brain Learns to Become Active in Bed

Does the following scenario sound familiar to you? "I was absolutely exhausted and could barely keep my eyes open. But when I got into bed, it was like a switch turned on, and I was wide awake." The scenario described is very common for those who have sleep problems. So, how is it that you can feel so sleepy outside of bed, but once in bed, you become completely awake? The answer may be your bed itself. Before you rush off to buy a new mattress, however, consider the following.

Animals, including humans, learn to associate stimuli (as Pavlov's dogs learned to associate the sound of a bell with the sight of food; see chapter 1) and can form very powerful associations between stimuli without intending to. Let's say you get food poisoning after eating at a restaurant. The next time you go to that restaurant, you may feel physically ill, even though the offending food is no longer there. Why does this happen? The answer is because unconsciously, you now associate the restaurant with feeling sick. Strong associations are formed in the presence of strong physical reactions, and that one experience was all it took for your body to link the restaurant with the following unpleasant involuntary response to the food. Your body identifies the restaurant, accurately or inaccurately, as one of the causes of your illness. The restaurant is now a cue for your body to feel sick. Associations that do not involve such a visceral response often require repeated similar experiences (or "pairings" of stimuli) to take effect, but the mechanism by which these associations are learned is more or less the same.

What does this have to do with an overactive mind in bed? Consider your bed as a stimulus. (In psychology, a stimulus is simply something that may or may not influence behavior, not necessarily something you would consider "stimulating"—though it can be.) If you have spent many nights tossing and turning in bed, or lying in bed while upset and unable to sleep, your bed has often been paired with tossing and turning, or being upset and not sleeping; perhaps your bed alone has become a cue for tossing and turning and being upset.

Turn Your Bed into a Cue for Sleep, Not Alertness

If your bed has become a cue for "switching on" alertness, anxiety, or frustration, you need to learn how to turn off the switch. Since repeated pairings of your bed with being awake and alert are the cause of the problem, you need to un-pair your bed with alertness and begin to pair it with sleep. To retrain your body and mind to rest instead of becoming active in bed, follow the six simple rules below. We have already mentioned the first four, but we will discuss them as they relate to retraining your body to be asleep in bed.

1. Do not nap.

2. Avoid wakeful activities in bed.

3. Be in bed only when asleep (or very close to sleep).

4. Get out of bed at the same time every day.

5. Get out of bed if unable to sleep.

6. Take your active mind out of bed.

Rule 1: *Do Not Nap*

Napping includes attempting to nap (unsuccessfully), dozing, or nodding off. The reason we ask you to refrain from napping is that you need to associate sleep with only one location (your bed) and one time (your sleep window). Dozing is usually an unintentional habit, so avoiding it takes some planning. Most people doze in a particular setting or at a particular time of day, for example while watching television in the evening. If you sometimes fall asleep by accident while watching television in the evening, use some preventative strategies: Do not lie down or recline on the furniture; sit up straight. Perhaps you can incorporate some light activity, such as folding laundry, while you watch television. If you live with someone, ask that person to help you stay awake.

Rule 2: *Avoid Wakeful Activities in Bed*

If you want your bed to become a strong cue for sleep rather than a cue for sleeplessness, your bed must be associated with sleep, not wakeful activities. So anything that you would normally do when awake should not occur in your bed. This includes using the computer, texting, talking on the phone, playing games, reading, watching television, eating, or any other activity that will signal wakefulness to your body in bed.

You may be wondering, *Does having sex count as a wakeful activity?* The answer to this question may depend upon how you typically feel about sex and after sex. Is sex, for you, an activity that is more often relaxing or invigorating? If after sex you feel sleepy, then perhaps sexual activity can be an exception to the rule. If after sex you feel alert (or if it is highly unpredictable whether you will feel alert after sex), you may want to explore having sex earlier in the day and in locations other than where you sleep. Or you may opt to make sex an exception to the rule anyway.

Many people have routines that they associate with relaxation, such as reading or watching television in bed. You may be reluctant to give up such habits. Here are a couple of things to keep in mind when deciding whether to make a change.

First, you may feel as if such habits help you relax; however, if you find yourself wide awake once the lights are turned off or once your head is on the pillow, then whatever relaxation you had is gone. Instead, you are now in a state of alertness. This is not to say that habits such as reading or watching television are not relaxing or that they need to be eliminated from your routine. Relaxation is an important part of getting a good night's sleep. Just move these habits out of the bed, and preferably out of the bedroom.

Second, you may not need to banish these activities forever. Given that you are reading this book, right now you probably experience sleep problems, but the tools we present will help rid you of them. When your sleep problems are under control, you may experiment with putting a previous habit back into your routine. (After all, you probably know people who read in bed yet sleep well. Perhaps as you begin to sleep well you will be able to join their ranks.) If you find that your sleep problems return, move wakeful activities back out of your bedroom and see whether your sleep improves again.

Rule 3: *Be in Bed Only When Asleep (or Very Close to Sleep)*

It makes sense that if your bed is to become a signal for sleep, you must pair it with sleep over and over again. The way to do this is to be in bed only when sleep is imminent. This means *go to bed only when you feel sleepy*. For many people with sleep problems, this advice is complicated because they often feel extremely tired but not *sleepy*. By sleepy, we mean "about to fall asleep." Feeling sleepy is different from feeling fatigued, feeling tired, or having low energy. By being in bed *only* when you are sleepy or asleep, you will un-train your body (and mind) from associating your bed with being awake and train it to associate your bed with sleeping.

It is possible that, when you first begin following this rule, you will have several nights of poor sleep. Fortunately, you have a natural system in your body that will make up for the sleep loss with deeper sleep (see chapter 3), and, ultimately, you will start sleeping better. You need to be strategic and be willing to accept a poor night or two, so that un-learning that your bed is associated with sleeplessness can happen and you can sleep better for many nights to come.

Rule 4: *Get Out of Bed at the Same Time Every Day*

If you want your body to know that when you are in bed, you should be asleep, you should set aside the same time each and every night for sleeping. However, because the rule above is that you are not to get into bed until your body feels *sleepy*, you may not always be able to control your bedtime. For example, your bedtime may be eleven, but if you do not feel sleepy at eleven, you must stay awake until you do. In contrast, you *can* control when you get out of bed in the morning, simply by setting an alarm. Setting an alarm becomes the anchor of your sleep period. Getting up at the same time each morning sets your body clock and also ensures that you are spending enough time out of bed to be building a drive for deep sleep. Moreover, if you get up at the same time each morning, seven days per week, you will start to become sleepy at around the same time every night. That is, your body will learn to produce sleep between certain hours of the night and *only* between those certain hours.

One thing to keep in mind is that in the beginning, when you follow rule 3 (be in bed only when asleep or very close to sleep), initially you may have some nights of poor sleep until your body gets the idea. However, it is very important that you get out of bed at your set rise time and resist the temptation to make up for lost sleep. Staying in bed past your usual rise time will have negative effects on your body clock, will prevent adequate buildup of drive for deep sleep, and will undermine the idea that sleep occurs only in your bed and only between certain hours. This will make it more likely that your body and mind will be wide awake the next night.

Rule 5: *Get Out of Bed If Unable to Sleep*

If you want your bed to be associated with sleep only, then you must get out of bed and preferably leave the room whenever it is obvious that you will not be able to fall asleep any time soon. We don't recommend you use a clock for this purpose, but you can usually tell within fifteen minutes of getting into bed whether you are going to have a hard time falling asleep.

What can you do when you leave the room? You can do anything that will not make you feel more awake. Pick an activity that is pleasurable or at least preferable to tossing and turning in bed, but one that does not make you feel more alert. Watching television in another room is a common and a good choice if the program you watch is not so engaging that you will be awake for the rest of the night watching it. Some people like to read, knit, or draw; others like to listen to music, a podcast, or an audiobook. Avoid activities that involve using very bright light and activities that are very engaging. Using the computer can be engaging and involve exposure to bright light— two elements that can increase how alert you feel—so we generally do not recommend it.

While awake in the middle of the night in a dark house, you must prioritize safety, so be sure that you have enough light to safely walk around. Ensuring safe lighting is of particular relevance for older adults and those on sleep medications. When you are in a different room and you start to feel sleepy, you can return to your room to sleep. If when you get into bed you become wide awake again, get out of bed again; be patient, as it may take some time for your body to get the message. It may take a few days, but your body will soon get the idea.

Rule 6: *Take Your Active Mind out of Bed*

Worrying, brooding, thinking, problem solving, mental list-making, and analyzing, even though they involve only your mind, are all activities that occur when you are awake, so they too can interfere with sleep and must be moved out of the bed. To train your mind to stop doing these activities in bed, get up and leave the bed, and preferably the bedroom; do not return to bed until these mental activities have quieted. You may find that these thoughts go away rather quickly or become less bothersome as soon as you leave the room. Getting out of bed when your mind is active may initially result in some poor nights, but eventually, either the mental activity in bed will decrease and/or the sleep deprivation will override the overactive mind; in either case, you will begin to sleep better.

Summary

This chapter explained specifically what you can do (some of which was also prescribed in previous chapters) to quiet your active nighttime mind that seems to maintain your sleep problems. The cause of an active mind when you want to sleep is often the type of learning called association, which may have taught your body through experience that your bed is a place where you do *not* sleep. Being in bed or staying in bed in the past when your mind was active may have led to your current problem of feeling awake and alert as soon as you get into bed. This happens unintentionally, of course, but you must actively work to undo this learning and retrain your body. You can do so by reducing or cutting out in-bed activities and getting out of bed whenever you are having trouble sleeping, thus preserving your bed as a sanctuary for sleeping (with the possible exception of sex). This will help you break the cycle of poor sleep in bed.

Chapter 5

Put a Buffer between the Day's Activity and Sleep

In order to prevent the day's unfinished business from interfering with sleep, we recommend you create a time each night that moves you away from the "active self" you are during the day and toward the "relaxed self" needed for sleeping. We call this time the Buffer Zone. You may believe that you take enough breaks in your day that you do not need a Buffer Zone; however, taking a break prior to getting ready for bed is almost always a necessity.

Do You Need a Buffer Zone?

Which of the following statements are often true for you?

- I think about problems in bed.

- I have trouble shutting my mind off at night.

- I become worried, tense, or anxious just before my bedtime.

- I worry in bed.

- I make to-do lists in my mind in bed.

- When I am in bed I find it difficult to resist the urge to check my e-mail or text messages or to answer the phone when it rings.

- I feel tense in bed.

- When I am in bed I think about things that have happened during the day.

These are all signs that you need to set aside time to deal with the day's business before getting into bed. In actuality, everyone probably needs a Buffer Zone.

What Can We Learn from Mr. Rogers?

Fred Rogers was an iconic late-twentieth-century children's television star who had a rather famous ritual during the opening of his show *Mister Rogers' Neighborhood*. Every single episode, he would walk in the door of his "home," take off his jacket and put on his trademark cardigan, then change out of his dress shoes into sneakers. In other words, when Mr. Rogers came home, there was a shift in his daily routine from a certain formality to relaxation and leisure. His time at home was spent interacting with friends, reading books, and enjoying his hobbies. This image of shifting gears in a deliberate way by changing your outfit may be helpful for you in coming up with your own Buffer Zone plan.

It may be that you lead a very busy life and your "work self" is constantly put upon to do difficult or stressful tasks. It is important to be able to make a distinction between that person—meaning your busy, goal-directed self—and your non-work self. Each day you should shift out of your busy, goal-directed self into a relaxed, winding-down self. Make this shift a part of your regular routine, and protect it; that is, try not to schedule activities that would conflict with the purpose of the Buffer Zone.

How to Establish a Buffer Zone

The Buffer Zone is a simple concept: it is a quiet time prior to bedtime. Every night, set aside time to do activities that promote rest and allow you to disengage from your busy life.

Prioritize Wind-Down Activities One Hour before Bedtime

To create a Buffer Zone, set aside an hour or so before bedtime during which you can do some calming, pleasant activities. This provides a transition between the goal-focused activities of the day and the quiet, more peaceful time of sleep. The activities you select for the Buffer Zone should be activities that are enjoyable in themselves and are not taken as a means to an end. Stay away from any activities that might be stimulating or that have the potential to upset you or cause you to worry.

Say "Good Night" to Your Personal Electronics

Many people use personal electronics to stay connected to their friends, family, and work. Even if you enjoy connecting to others through your personal electronic devices, social activity close to bedtime can interfere with the process of disconnecting from your active life and the day's excitement and tensions so that sleep can unfold naturally. Waiting for the next text or e-mail, thinking of a response, and then waiting for the next message to arrive can create a sense of alertness that can interfere with sleep. Additionally, for some people, using personal electronics becomes addictive. If you became tense when you read the heading "Say 'Good Night' to Your Personal Electronics," it may be useful to examine why this thought makes you tense. Anxiety drives compulsive behavior, and anxiety is not conducive to sleep. The best way to get rid of a compulsive behavior is to resist doing it and engage in an alternative behavior that is incompatible with the behavior you want to change. For example, turn off your personal device—your cell phone, portable gaming device, or tablet—and leave it in a different room (so that it is not handy) while you engage in something enjoyable and calming. Pretty soon, you will develop the habit of powering down your devices at night, and you may find yourself less alert close to bedtime. Later in this chapter you will find a list of activities you might consider for your Buffer Zone.

Adjusting the Duration of Your Buffer Zone

Although the rule of thumb is to institute an hour-long Buffer Zone, for people who have difficulty staying awake in the evening, an hour may be too long. This may be a particular problem for early birds (those who become sleepy early and rise early). If you find yourself nodding off in the evening, shorten your Buffer Zone to thirty minutes.

On the other hand, a variety of things can make it necessary to have a longer Buffer Zone. Your day may have been unusually active and stressful, or your evening activity may have been very exciting or upsetting; on such evenings, an hour may not provide enough time for you to distance yourself from the day's excitement. People who are night owls are more prone to becoming alert late in the evening and may require a longer Buffer Zone and very careful attention to the type of activities they select for it. In general, if you find that you are frequently unable to disengage from the day even after an hour of unwinding, consider lengthening your Buffer Zone.

However, one hour is usually plenty of time for a wind-down period. If you are tempted to have your Buffer Zone start the moment you return home from work, or if you begin avoiding evening activities—such as socializing, housework, or hobbies—because you are worried they will interfere with sleep, you may be too worried about your sleep. Your life may have become just about working and sleeping, or more accurately *not* sleeping. Living this way is not helpful for sleep and may increase your vulnerability to depression. There is a difference between engaging in activities that help you wind down from a busy day and avoiding engaging in normal activities. The former can promote sleep; the latter can mean that you are preoccupied with sleep, and that could backfire and interfere with sleep.

Possible Buffer Zone Activities

The best activities for the Buffer Zone—your transition time—are those that are done for the sake of enjoyment and are not goal-oriented. We recommend that you create a list of appropriate activities to choose from during your Buffer Zone; below are some ideas to get you started. Keep in mind, however, that what may be a good Buffer Zone activity for one person may not be so good for another person, because people differ in how they approach certain activities. For example, many people enjoy solitaire, yet some play mindlessly just to pass the time while others strive to break a record time or a record score. For the former sort of player, solitaire is likely calming and a good Buffer Zone activity, but for the latter it may generate high levels of alertness.

- Reading a book

- Listening to music or a podcast

- Watching television

- Taking a bath/shower/sauna

- Doing yoga or tai chi

- Looking at a magazine or a book with art/photographs

- Playing a musical instrument

- Drawing or painting

- Watching sports

- Crafting

- Playing billiards or other games

- Knitting

- Stargazing

- Meditating

"I Have Too Many Responsibilities to Create a Buffer Zone."

If you cannot imagine establishing a Buffer Zone because you are busy meeting the needs of everyone around you right up until the moment you get into bed, it may be time to assess whether *you yourself* should become a higher priority in your life. You may be Super-Mom or Super-Dad, Super-Friend, Super-Wife or Super-Husband, Super-Employee, or Super-Boss, but if you play this role to the exclusion of your own needs, you may become your own archenemy.

You may have convinced yourself that you do not require leisure or rest, but all human beings have needs, and these needs cannot come second to everyone else's needs without a cost. At a minimum, the cost is poor sleep, but you can also expect other negative health consequences. If you do not take care of yourself, you will have less to give to others. Consider some of the following strategies, designed to help you to start to prioritize your own health and well-being:

- Think of the needs of the people who currently depend upon you. Now think of your own needs. Is your list of needs shorter? If so, why? How are your needs different from theirs? Why are you an exception? What is missing from your list of needs? Add to your list of needs and make time to de-stress and unwind every single night.

- Know that you will be more effective at providing help to people who depend on you if you make it a priority to take care of yourself.

- Remind yourself that everyone needs a break daily.

- Say no to at least one request this week.

- Set limits with those who demand too much of you.

- Let people know that you are making a change in your life and that, except for emergencies, you are unavailable each night starting at _____ o'clock.

If you are concerned that you will have trouble implementing a Buffer Zone because you find it difficult to disengage from work, it may be time to assess whether your relationship with work is potentially harmful. An imbalance between your work life and your personal life may be behind your sleep problems. Are you obsessed with work to the exclusion of other things in your life? Some people work as though they were addicted to working. Have you convinced yourself that you have to work harder than everyone else? At your place of work, are you always the first to arrive and the last to leave? Has anyone ever accused you of being a workaholic or a perfectionist? Do you feel as if you are addicted to work? Work and your professional identity may be overly tied to your self-esteem so that you over-allocate time to work pursuits. Do you feel badly about yourself when you are not doing work? Do you view non-work activities as a waste of time? Do you believe that any idle time should be filled with some *useful* activity toward a goal? Have you come to devalue activities done for the sake of leisure or rest? If so, here are some things for you to try:

- Ask yourself, *Why am I the exception to the rule that human beings need rest and relaxation?* In other words, challenge the idea that you do not require rest or pleasure in your life—all human beings do.

- Imagine what would happen at work if you were incapacitated in some way. Would the business cease to exist, or would it find some way to make up for your absence? Challenge your tendency to overestimate your importance at work. Paradoxically, people who take breaks and recharge are often more productive at work.

- Experiment with putting some rest and pleasure into your life and taking away some of the time currently allotted to work. For example, if you are working more than eight hours a day, commit to leaving work at an earlier time this week. Spend that extra time doing something enjoyable.

- Shorten your to-do list this week to essentials only.

- In your own personal currency (i.e., in your mind), consider increasing the value of moments of pleasure and decreasing the value of accomplishments.

Summary

Like any other human being, you need time for rest and relaxation. This chapter explained how having a Buffer Zone can help your mind prepare for sleep by putting the day's activities and worries behind you. It is easy to create a Buffer Zone: about an hour before getting ready for bed, begin to transition away from your "active self" by restricting your activities to those that are relaxing and enjoyable to you. Taking this time for yourself and leaving behind work or personal responsibilities at the end of the day will help you get a better night's sleep so that you can be at your best tomorrow. Far from being wasted time, a Buffer Zone will help you be more productive in your "on" hours.

Chapter 6

Relax Your Body to Quiet Your Mind

The previous chapter provided strategies for winding down so that you can leave the day's excitement and tension behind. Although setting time aside to unwind is essential, sometimes setting time aside is not enough to produce relaxation and you may need a deliberate strategy; that is, an active relaxation practice. If you find yourself tense or anxious, starting a formal relaxation practice may be just the solution for you. There is reason to think that a relaxation practice alone may help those with sleep problems, but if you combine a relaxation practice with the other strategies in this book you will see a more thorough improvement in your sleep.

"Just Relax"?

Are you particularly tense and anxious at night? Are you frustrated by your seeming inability to relax? Just as difficulty sleeping makes many people anxious, difficulty relaxing can produce anxiety. Perhaps you have already tried relaxation for your sleep problems and felt more anxious because you were unable to relax. Even if relaxation did not seem to work for you in the past, it does not mean a relaxation practice cannot benefit you at all. You simply need to keep the following keys to success in mind.

Practice, Practice, Practice

The ability to relax is a skill and, like any other skill, it requires practice to attain. Learning to relax is like learning to play the piano: you will not be a virtuoso after one lesson. Similarly, you cannot expect to sleep soundly on the first few nights you practice relaxation. You are retraining your body and building a skill. Setting unrealistic expectations will lead you to quit prematurely.

In his book *Full Catastrophe Living*, Jon Kabat-Zinn, PhD, a renowned expert in stress management, suggested that starting a practice, such as a relaxation practice, is like weaving a parachute (1990). You would never choose to start weaving your parachute when you are already falling—you would want it done in advance. In other words, relaxation strategies must be learned and practiced ahead of time, so that when you are in an anxious state, you are able to simply pull the rip cord of your relaxation parachute and begin to relax. So commit to practicing a relaxation strategy daily for several weeks, and you will be amazed by the result.

You may be worried that your body *cannot* relax, but this is exactly why you need to practice. Even if you believe that your body is incapable of relaxing, you can notice subtle changes in your sensation of muscle tension if you pay close attention. Your body's relaxation system is not "broken"; it just needs a tune-up. The tune-up process starts with observing the difference between how it feels when your muscles are deliberately clenched and the sensation of releasing that tension. By focusing on the difference between these two opposing states, you will see that you *can* relax, at least to some degree. With practice, and patience, it will be easier for you to relax, and your sensations of relaxation will grow deeper.

Relax about Relaxation

There have been many different tests of one form of relaxation versus another in helping people overcome sleep problems, with no clear winners. You should thus feel free to explore different methods of relaxation, seeing which methods feel best to you. Approach relaxation with a curious and open mind-set. (Different relaxation strategies are described later in this chapter.) Relax your expectations, because in the beginning it is more about learning than achieving any specific state of relaxation.

Practice When You Are Awake

Often, people try to practice relaxation in bed, in hopes that it will act like a sleeping pill, but this is not likely to be effective and may be frustrating and discouraging. To be effective in bed, relaxation needs to first be learned outside of bed, through practice and focused attention. You will know that you are ready to start using relaxation in bed when you notice that you can transition into a state of relaxation during your daytime practice.

Learn How to Step on Your Body's Anxiety Brakes

Although you may not like anxiety, you could not survive without it. In an emergency situation, anxiety grabs your attention and allows you to respond either by fleeing the situation or by summoning extra resources so that your body can manage the emergency. The human body has complementary systems that control physical activation and deactivation as well as relaxation and tension. You can think of this system as similar to a car's brake and gas pedals. To drive, you need both the gas and the brakes. In your body, the "gas" is the *sympathetic* nervous system, and the "brakes" are the *parasympathetic* nervous system.

When you need to move in a hurry (as in an emergency), your sympathetic nervous system becomes active and your heart rate increases, you start to breathe more quickly, more blood flows to your large muscles (in your arms and legs), and physical functions that can be postponed, such as digestion, are temporarily put on hold. This is like stepping on the gas. This is the system that helps you when you need to run away from or directly face a threat, such as an intruder. This system is also active even when the danger you perceive is not a "true" or immediate emergency. For example, if you are feeling anxious about something that may never happen or will not happen for several days, this system can still become active and produce sensations of alertness, tension, and anxiety.

Naturally, it is unwise to sleep if you perceive danger. In other words, the sensations produced by an overactive sympathetic nervous system in response to a real or imagined danger are not conducive to sleep. You cannot sleep when your sympathetic nervous system is overactive: you first need the parasympathetic nervous system to step on the brakes. When the parasympathetic nervous system is activated, your heart rate decreases, your breathing slows, the blood flows evenly throughout your body, and important physical functions such as digestion resume. It is a system responsible for rest and restoration. If you were to learn how to step on your brakes at will, you would have a powerful tool at bedtime and would no longer be bothered by a noisy mind in bed.

Make a Plan for Relaxation This Week

Making a change in your routine can be difficult. The easiest way to maintain a change in behavior is to make a plan for how it can become a habit. Now that you know that chronic tension may underlie your insomnia and that managing this tension requires practice, it is important to prioritize this practice over the next few weeks. Look at your current schedule and set aside at least twenty minutes per day for this practice. Over the coming weeks, keep track of how often you are actually able to stick to this commitment. On days that you did not stick to this commitment, what got in the way? Take some time to understand why you did not do it. Do not criticize yourself for not engaging in your relaxation practice; instead, set aside some time to troubleshoot what went wrong and how you may be able to make an adjustment.

The most common obstacle to making relaxation a habit is a perceived lack of time. If you do not have twenty minutes in your day to attend to your health, you are likely overscheduled and this may be the source of your tension and noisy mind at night. Once you have made some time in your schedule, try to arrange some time in which you will not be interrupted. Put away your personal electronics and/or set your phone to silent. If you have children, arrange for child care or engage in this practice after your children go to bed. Tell your spouse, partner, or roommate that you are embarking on a relaxation program and would appreciate some quiet time each evening. Make a change over the next month and see the benefits of a relaxation practice.

Relaxation Strategies

As we mentioned, no particular relaxation strategy is better than another, so try out a variety of strategies and determine which ones suit you best. You can create a list of relaxation strategies to try over the next few weeks. Below, we provide a few tested strategies, but keep in mind that many more exist. There are many other self-help books, such as *The Relaxation and Stress Reduction Workbook* by Martha Davis, Elizabeth Robbins Eshelman, and Matthew McKay (New Harbinger Publications, 2008), that are devoted to relaxation strategies.

Progressive Muscle Relaxation

Progressive muscle relaxation (PMR) is a very commonly used relaxation technique. This exercise will teach you the difference in sensation in each muscle group between holding muscle tension and then releasing the tension; that is, muscle relaxation.

The instructions below will walk you through the exercise. Because PMR is meant to be done with the eyes closed, the italicized passages can be your script if you wish to make a recording to guide you. Take your time with each muscle group, and pause for about fifteen seconds or more between each muscle group. Or you can use the recording of this exercise at author Colleen Carney's Ryerson University web page: ryerson.ca/~ccarney/. There are also many CDs on the market that will guide you through PMR.

As with any relaxation practice, start by finding a comfortable position, either seated or lying down. Take a deep breath, hold it for a few moments and then slowly exhale. Prepare your mind for a practice focused only in the here and now. You are devoting this time to paying attention to your body and learning the sensation of the release of muscle tension.

Bring your awareness to your right foot. Tense the muscles in your foot by pointing and curling your toes as you turn your foot inward. Hold the tension in your foot. Notice how it feels to tense your entire foot. Hold for ten seconds. Now as you release the tension and relax your foot, focus all of your attention on the sensation of the release of this tension. Notice how different it feels from when the muscles in your foot were tensed. Let your foot relax very deeply. You may notice a warming or tingling sensation in your foot. Take fifteen seconds to continue focusing on the different sensation now that you have released the tension.

Note that you do not have to be 100 percent relaxed in order for this to be effective. Accept that in the beginning you may still hold some tension. PMR is about perceptually learning the difference between the two sensations. After fifteen seconds, switch to the left foot and repeat the process. (If you are making a recording, repeat the above passage, simply changing "right" to "left.")

Once you have tensed and relaxed both feet, and paused for fifteen seconds, move on to the next muscle group.

Now bring your awareness to your right calf or the muscles in your lower leg. Tense these muscles by pulling your toes toward your head and notice how it feels when the calf is tensed. Now hold the muscle tension and your focus on this area for ten seconds. Now relax your calf and notice the difference in sensation from when the muscles were tensed. Focus your awareness on how relaxed the calf feels in comparison to when it was tense.

After fifteen seconds, focusing on the sensation of relaxation, repeat the process with your left calf. (If you are making a recording, repeat the above passage, simply changing "right" to "left.")

Pause for fifteen seconds or more, and when you are ready, bring your attention to your right upper leg. To tense these muscles, you can try to straighten your leg while at the same time trying to bend your leg at the knee—but do not actually move your leg. Focus on the opposing actions of the two muscles working against each other.

Note: If your muscles cramp or spasm during any of the tension components of this exercise, you are exerting too much force. You merely need to produce some tension.

Focus on the tension in your upper leg and thigh. Notice the tightness in your leg muscles and hold for ten seconds. Now release the tension in your upper leg and focus on the sensation of release. Notice how different your leg feels as you relax it. Let it relax very deeply, and when it feels very relaxed, pause for about fifteen seconds.

Then repeat the process for your left thigh.

Now turn your attention to your hip and buttock area. Flex your buttock muscles and the sides of your hips. Focus your attention on this part of the body and the sensation produced by the flexion. If you are able, hold the tension for at least ten seconds. Now focus your attention on the release of these muscles. Notice the difference in sensation between the tension and the release. Focus your attention for at least fifteen more seconds on this part of your body.

Now focus on your stomach area. You will tense your stomach muscles by making your stomach as hard as you can make it. Notice how tight the area feels as you tense your stomach. Try to hold the tension for at least ten seconds. Now, relax your stomach and notice the release of air from your stomach and the release of your stomach muscles. Notice the difference between tension and relaxation as you let go of the tension in your stomach. Continue to focus on this sensation in your stomach for about fifteen seconds.

Now, focus your attention on the muscles in your upper torso. You will tense these muscles by inhaling and pulling your shoulder blades together. Do not exert too much force. Notice how it feels when your upper back and shoulders are tensed. Hold for ten seconds. Now exhale and release those muscles. Let go of all of the tension and notice how different that feels. Continue to focus on this area for another fifteen seconds.

Now, focus your attention on your upper right arm. Tense this area by bending your arm at the elbow and bringing your hand up toward your shoulder. Tense your bicep and study how the tension feels. Hold this tension for about ten seconds.

Note: As with every muscle group, if you feel pain or experience a spasm, ease up on the tension. You need only focus on the sensation of how holding tension in your muscles feels.

Now release the tension and notice how different the tension and relaxation feel. Continue to relax your bicep and focus on the sensation of relaxation for another fifteen seconds. Now move your attention a little farther down your arm, to the muscles in your hand and forearm. You can tighten these muscles by making a tight fist and holding it. Focus your attention on how the tension feels in this area of your body. After about ten seconds, relax your hand and forearm by opening your fist, letting your fingers unfurl effortlessly. As you do so, notice the sensations in your hand and forearm. Notice how the tension feels different from the relaxation. Continue to relax your hand and forearm and study the sensations for another fifteen seconds.

Repeat the preceding portion of the exercise for your left arm.

Having tensed and relaxed the muscles in your hands and arms, you can now move up to your neck. You can tense these muscles by pulling your chin toward your chest and at the same time keep it from touching your chest. Hold this tension for about ten seconds and focus all of your attention on the sensation of tension in your neck. Now release your neck muscles and focus your attention on the sensation of release. If you are lying down, allow your head to gently sink toward the floor, releasing all tension in your neck. Notice the difference between the sensations of relaxation and tension. Hold your focus on your relaxed neck muscles for about fifteen seconds.

Now move the focus of your attention to the muscles of your lower face. You can tense these muscles by biting down and, at the same time, pulling back the corners of your mouth. Hold the tension for at least ten seconds and really focus on how it feels to tighten these muscles. Now, as you relax the muscles and allow the corners of your mouth to fall forward, notice the difference between tension and relaxation. Continue to focus for another fifteen seconds on the relaxed muscles of your lower face. It does not matter whether your face is 100 percent relaxed. It is more important to notice the difference between tension and relaxation and focus on the sensation of release. In time and with practice, your relaxation will deepen.

Now focus your attention on the muscles in the central part of your face. You will tense these muscles by squinting (narrowing your eyes) as tightly as you can and simultaneously wrinkling your nose. Tense these muscles now, focusing on how the tension feels. Feel the tightness and hold for ten seconds. Now let go of the tension in your face. Notice how it feels to release the tension and allow your eye muscles to soften and fall back into place and to *allow the sides of your nose to soften and fall back into a relaxed state. Continue to relax these muscles for fifteen more seconds.*

Last, focus on the muscles in your upper face. You will tense these muscles by raising your eyebrows as high as possible. Tense these muscles now. Feel the tightness in your upper face and focus on this sensation for about ten seconds. Now, relax your upper face; let your eyebrows drop, and feel the tension releasing from this area. Continue to relax and focus on the difference in sensation from the tension for about fifteen seconds.

With mastery of this exercise, you will be able to merely scan your body for any particular areas of tension and then release that tension.

Guided Imagery

You may experience anxiety as pictures of upsetting scenes flashing through your mind, along with sensations of fear such as a racing heart. For example, you may picture a scene of getting fired at work and wake up with your heart pounding. Many people find it useful to focus on imagery that can neutralize anxiety or even create opposite sensations such as relaxation and a state of peace and calm. Although it may take some practice, this kind of exercise may be very useful for you in teaching yourself to create a calming state. As with most relaxation practices, try to set aside at least twenty minutes a day.

The idea of guided imagery is to imagine a pleasant, calming scene. Below is a guided imagery exercise for a beach scene. You can adapt it to any scene you find particularly soothing. Do not restrict yourself to places you have been; feel free to imagine a place you've never visited or even one of your own invention. You may even enjoy a fantasy scene in which you are floating through the sky. If you create your own scene, describe it as vividly as possible and include as many of the five senses in your description as possible. Describe sights, sounds, smells, textures, and, if relevant, tastes too. We recommend that you make an audio recording, whether you are describing your own scene or reading the scene below, so that you can listen to it with your eyes closed during this exercise. Most people find it easier to focus on mental images if their eyes are closed.

THE BEACH

Lie down or get into whatever position is comfortable for you. Take a deep breath to mark the start of your practice. Slow your breathing down. Close your eyes to help you focus on slowing your breathing down and bringing your attention to the present moment. Scan through your body. Bring awareness to any areas that are currently tense. Breathe deeply, and imagine the breath flowing into whatever areas of your body seem tense. As you slow your breathing, in the distance you hear a seagull calling. In your mind's eye, you look around and notice you are on a long stretch of the most beautiful white sand beach you have ever seen. The sun overhead feels warm on your face. Take a moment to just focus on the warmth. What does it feel like? What do you hear? What do you smell at the beach? The breeze is gently blowing through your hair. You take a deep breath of the salty sea air and close your eyes. The bright sun is peeking through your closed eyelids. Focus on the sensation of the warm sand beneath your feet. Look down and see your foot in the sand. Focus on the sensation. When you are ready, slowly start walking and focus on the sensation of the sole of your foot spreading deeper into the sand, the grains of sand filling the spaces between your toes. Feel the sensation as you roll up onto your toes and you step down with your other foot into the sand. Look back at your footprints behind you. Hear the gentle crashing of the waves. The waves are mesmerizing, as there is a rhythm to the tide. You feel yourself becoming more and more relaxed with every wave. Take a few moments to focus on the sound and sight of the waves and how each one brings you closer to relaxation. Imagine sitting on the sandy beach. Watch the waves for a moment. Feel your seat sinking into the soft sand, forming the perfect chair beneath you. The water is clear, and the tips of the waves are foamy and white. You see tiny fish swimming in the water. The sun is now low in the sky, and against the beautiful blue sky are orange, gold, yellow, and pink colors. You are again aware of the warmth on your face and arms. If there is any tension in your body, focus the warmth on the tense area and breathe warm air into it. You are in a state of calm and serenity. Stay here in your scene as long as you want.

Belly Breathing

Take a moment right now to observe your breathing. When you are calm, your breathing is deep and slow and often emanates from your belly. When you are anxious or tense, your breathing is quick and shallow and comes from your chest. Breathing from your belly, also called diaphragmatic breathing, can help you transition into a deeper state of relaxation. It takes some practice, but it is very effective at producing relaxation throughout your body and mind.

To begin, find a comfortable position. If you are comfortable sitting, shift in your seat to find an even more comfortable position but try to have your back straight. If you are lying down, shift until you find a comfortable spot. Put one hand on your chest and the other on your stomach. You may find the sensation of resting your hands on your belly and chest comforting. Now, breathe in through your nose directly to the stomach. The hand on your stomach should rise. The hand on your chest should move very little. This may seem strange, and it may take a few breaths to coordinate the inhalation with your belly filling and rising. When you exhale, exhale through your mouth, pushing out as much air as you can while contracting your abdominal muscles. The hand on your stomach should move in as you exhale, but your other hand should move very little. Continue to breathe in through your nose and out through your mouth. Try to inhale enough so that your lower abdomen rises and falls. Count slowly as you exhale.

You may find it most relaxing when you are able to inhale for a slow count of three, hold for a count of three, and exhale for a count of three. Doing so will slow down your breathing, and when your breathing is slow, the rest of your body will feel more relaxed. Do this for as long as you like. Practice consistently; set aside about twenty minutes to do this exercise daily. Eventually, you will be able to scan your body and readily detect when your breathing is shallow and correct it by slowing down your breathing and entering a state of relaxation. However, this will take considerable practice.

Yoga

There are many benefits to a yoga practice, such as increased flexibility, decreased pain, increased stamina and fitness, and, of course, relaxation. There are different types of yoga, including practices designed to strengthen your body and increase your energy. Two of the more common yoga practices for purposes of relaxation are Satyananda yoga and Hatha yoga. If you will be taking one of several classes offered by the same instructor, the instructor can recommend the class most suited for a relaxation practice. If you prefer to use a DVD or some other self-directed means of practicing yoga, be sure to read the description of the practice to look for key words like "relaxation."

Yoga may be a good practice for you because it combines breathing, muscle relaxation, and imagery, described above. As with any relaxation practice, commit to practicing for at least a short while every day, but set your expectations low for the first several weeks. If you are too attached to the idea of instant and deep relaxation, you may become frustrated quickly and give up before you are able to reap the rewards of these practices.

Other Relaxation Practices

The choices for relaxation are endless. Enjoy exploring all the other forms of relaxation available to you. These may include:

- Tai chi

- Relaxation sounds or music CDs

- Massage

- Chanting (e.g., "ohm")

- Meditation

- Warm baths

Summary

In this chapter, you learned that you can address the problem of a noisy mind by learning to quiet your body, or reduce muscle tension. When your sympathetic nervous system is activated because of perceived danger—when your body is "stepping on the gas"—the resulting increased heart rate, quickened breathing, and so on make it difficult to sleep. By practicing relaxation techniques, you can figuratively step on the brakes when you wish to reduce your tension and anxiety.

In this chapter, we described progressive muscle relaxation, belly breathing, imagery, and yoga, but these are not the only strategies you may use. Choose which technique or techniques work best for you, and try to make time to practice every day. If you are careful to have reasonable expectations, you will find that after a while sleep does come more easily.

Chapter 7

Manage Your Overactive Mind without Counting Sheep

You may be reading this book because you want a strategy for counteracting the frustrating experience of lying awake worrying. Hopefully you have learned from the preceding chapters that multiple factors can contribute to bedtime worrying and that there are things you can do to make your sleep system run optimally and make bedtime worrying less likely. In this chapter, you will read about strategies to "put your worries to bed" so that you can have a more restful sleep.

Put Your Worries to Bed

Do you have a busy life? Do you remain so busy throughout your day that you have the chance to think about what is happening in your life only when you get into bed, a place that is quiet and dark and free of distractions?

When you are half asleep, you are not at your problem-solving best and you may be even more prone to imagining unlikely disasters and worrying about things over which you have little control. The solution? Problem solve intentionally at a time when you are better able to generate good solutions. Give yourself a time to address your worries earlier in the day so that bedtime is no longer your only available time to think about the day's events.

Schedule a Worry Time

If you give yourself time earlier in the day to deal with unfinished business, your worries will be less likely to follow you to bed. Start by scheduling a time in the early evening when you can have about twenty to thirty minutes of uninterrupted time. Divide a sheet of paper (or an electronic document) in half by drawing a vertical line down the middle. At the top of the left-hand column write "Worries or Concerns." Label the right-hand column "Next Steps" or "Solutions."

What typically worries you at night? Is there something on your mind right now that may bother you later? Do you have a problem for which you have not yet thought of a solution? These are all good candidates for your "Worries or Concerns" column. Once you have recorded a worry, think of the next step you could take toward resolution. Try to think of several possible solutions for each problem. Once you have generated several solutions, focus on the best "next" step that you can take. For example, if your worry is that you have a bill that is due soon and you are not sure whether it was paid, ultimately the solution is to pay it if it remains outstanding; however, there are intervening steps that you should write down. For example, you will need to look on the computer or wherever you track your bill payments to see whether the bill was paid. This is just a small step toward paying the bill, but it makes the process more manageable.

Most people who worry can generate good solutions to problems; however, their problems seem so overwhelming that they fail to actually take steps to solve them. Breaking a solution or a goal down into smaller steps increases the likelihood that you will move toward it. You may find that accomplishing the first small step inspires you to move to the next step, helping you meet your goal. If you have several unmet goals, you may be prone to feeling anxious, frustrated, or even depressed. Try breaking them down and working on them in this way, and you may feel better.

You may choose to work on only one worry per day, or you may use your worry time to generate a "to-do" list to solve mini-worries. Simply take time to work on whatever problems come up.

Some problems may not have immediate solutions or may be entirely out of your control. When a solution cannot be immediately pursued, thinking about possible solutions and making plans for different scenarios may help you feel less stuck. If the problem is entirely out of your control, however, constructive solutions are not realistic. In this case, it helps to just write about the problem and accept that a solution is not within your control. Let's say you are looking for a job. You have already created a plan for identifying and applying for jobs, worked on your CV, and done everything else that you possibly can. Yet you are still worried about getting a job. At this point, things are out of your control and it is best to focus on taking care of yourself so that you maintain the energy and optimism to wait until one of your job prospects pays off. Sometimes actively reassuring yourself that things will be okay is the next best step to resolving a worry. If worries about finding a job persist, do some free writing about them.

When your worry time is up, fold the paper in half and put it away. Reassure yourself that you have done the best that you can do for now. Re-remind yourself of this if the worry intrudes into your nighttime routine. That is, remind yourself that you already dealt with the problem when you were at your problem-solving best earlier in the evening and there is nothing that you can do about it now, when it is time to sleep.

Write about Your Concerns at Bedtime

Some people find that, despite their earlier evening problem solving, they worry again at bedtime. You may find that writing before you go to sleep helps you let these things go and allows you to fall asleep more readily. This strategy allows you to organize your thoughts about something that is on your mind, process it, and then let it go.

As before, set aside twenty to thirty minutes for this purpose. Start by writing down thoughts, concerns, or simply things on your mind. Be as honest as possible, openly exploring your deepest feelings and thoughts about matters that bother you. Some people find it easier to write openly if they plan to shred their writing when they are done. Include as much detail as possible and freely explore every aspect of what you are writing about. Do not censor yourself or tell yourself that your thoughts are too "silly" to put down on paper; whatever you write about is okay. Once you have completely explored the topic, put your paper away (shred it if you wish).

Do this whenever you find yourself worried before or in bed.

Banish Worry from Your Bed

If you worry in bed, it may become an unwanted habit and you will be more likely to continue to worry in the future. Below are some tips that will make it less likely for worry to occur while you are trying to sleep.

Get Out of Bed

Worrying in bed may have several causes. Perhaps bedtime represents your first opportunity to process the day's events, because during the day you either pushed your thoughts away or were too busy to think about things. Perhaps your bed has become a place where you struggle night after night and therefore you approach bed feeling alert or anxious. In this state of mind, you are more likely to start thinking about things that worry you.

Whatever the reason, worrying in bed can become a habit. One of the most effective ways to break this habit is to get out of bed once the worrying starts. This strategy is described in full in chapter 4; however, we will review the rationale here as it pertains to worrying in bed. If your bed has become associated with worrying, problem solving, list-making, or ruminating about things that went wrong in your day, you need to protect your bed from being paired with these unwanted mental habits. To do so, get out of bed and go to another room until this mental activity (worrying, problem solving, list-making, or ruminating) subsides.

It is possible that when you first start to use this strategy you will spend a lot of time out of bed at night and sleep even less, but this will be a short-term side effect and a relatively small price to pay for solving the problem in the long run. The sleep deprivation that may result from getting out of bed when unable to sleep will increase your sleep drive (the pressure to sleep), and if you do it consistently you will quickly start sleeping better. Your bed will be associated with sleep rather than worry, and as a result you can expect improved sleep for many more nights in the future.

A rule of thumb is if you worry for what feels like longer than fifteen minutes (do not watch the clock) or if you are feeling wide awake in bed, it is best to leave the room and not return to bed until you are sleepy and not worrying.

Occupy Your Mind

Racing thoughts and a tense body make it difficult for you to have restful sleep. You may try to deal with this problem by trying to force yourself to feel less anxious; in other words, you may simply try to will yourself to stop worrying.

We would like you to do the following exercise: When you reach the end of this paragraph, close your eyes and try *not* to think about a banana split. Do not imagine the cold ice cream. Do not imagine the scent of banana. Do not think of the chocolate syrup drizzling on the top. Do not picture how the sweet juice bursts out of the maraschino cherry as you bite into it. Also do not think, *I will not think of banana splits.* After all, thinking of the absence of a banana split also constitutes thinking of banana splits.

You get the picture. The answer to this conundrum is to find alternatives to "stopping" unwanted thoughts from occurring. We will discuss several, and in a later chapter we will discuss the power of being open to the experience. First we discuss the strategy of finding something compelling to occupy your mind.

Have you ever been told to count sheep to help you fall asleep? Try this little experiment right now. Sit comfortably and close your eyes. Imagine a field with a single fence. What does your fence look like? What color is it? How high is it? Is it made of wood? Does it stretch the entire vista of your mind? Or is it only one or two sections of fence? Once you have a clear vision of what the fence looks like, imagine a sheep approaching the fence and jumping effortlessly and slowly over the fence. As the sheep's front feet touch the grass on the other side, a second sheep jumps with exactly the same height and velocity. As the second sheep's feet touch the ground on the other side, a third sheep begins the jump. Watch a fourth sheep jump. And a fifth sheep. And a sixth sheep. All of your sheep jump with the same form, speed, height, and arc. And then a seventh sheep jumps. And an eighth. A ninth and a tenth. Then open your eyes and read on.

What did you notice? Some people find the monotony of this visual experiment relaxing and notice nothing except the image of the sheep jumping. Others are distracted by thoughts during the exercise. Perhaps you had thoughts such as "This would never work at night" or "This is boring," or perhaps you thought of other things that were on your mind.

What does the sheep exercise tell us? Engaging your mind in an exercise in which you picture something in your mind's eye occupies space in your busy mind. However, this exercise also tells us that if the picture is boring, you may become distracted by unrelated thoughts. In other words, there is a strategy here: engage your mind in a visual image that will compete with other thoughts. Perhaps sheep jumping over a fence isn't quite engaging enough to hold the attention of your overactive mind, particularly in a dark, quiet bedroom. What, then, may work better?

Consider the human fondness for stories. Many of the things people like to do to unwind involve following a storyline. People generally seek out stories—whether told on the radio, in a book, on television, or in some other form—for diversion and entertainment. You may be surprised to learn that there is a way you can enjoy stories in bed without using your eyes or ears.

Tonight when you get into bed, think about a story with particularly compelling characters or a fascinating plot. It can be a story from a book, a movie, a television show, a play, or your imagination. Follow the plot from whatever point you like. You may like to imagine what happens after the end of a favorite movie or book. Or you may like to come up with an alternate ending. If you have a vivid imagination, you may imagine a completely new story for a character you find compelling. The only rule is to avoid selecting a story that is likely to be so exciting that it would keep you awake. You want something that will hold your interest more than sheep jumping over a fence, but not so much that you become wide awake. Be sure to focus on the details in your imagined scenes. Details help make the image vivid and engaging. What are people wearing? What are they saying? What does the room or setting look like? Focus on what would happen next. Occupy your mind and enjoy the story you create. If you find it difficult to think of a story, you may like to incorporate a hobby. For example, imagine that you are decorating a home room by room on an unlimited budget or that you are golfing a perfect game on a fantasy course. As long as it is not too exciting, it doesn't matter what you visualize.

Challenge Worries about Sleeplessness

Is your worry specifically about sleep or sleeplessness? If so, you may have already realized that thinking about being sleepless makes you anxious. You may have found that your anxiety and frustration make it even more likely that you will think about how worried you are about sleeplessness, making you more anxious and sleep even more elusive. One way to interrupt this cycle of worrying is to challenge the idea that being sleepless is a complete disaster.

When you find yourself awake in the middle of the night, do any of the following thoughts occur?

- *This is horrible!*

- *I can't take it!*

- *I need to get to sleep now, or I'm going to have a horrible day.*

Consider a seemingly silly question for a moment: what is so inherently bad about being awake? Try the following exercise: write down "Being awake at night is a complete disaster because…." Then list all the reasons you can come up with, even those that may seem silly as you write them; no one has to see this list. Now consider how having these thoughts affects your sleep. Are there any consequences to having these thoughts? Answer this question for each of the items on your list.

Imagine two people, Anne and Janet, each with a different reaction to being awake at 2:00 a.m. Anne thinks: *Oh my god—it's 2:00 a.m. If I don't fall asleep within the next twenty minutes, I am going to lose it.* Janet thinks: *Ugh, it's 2:00 a.m.—I might as well go watch television rather than lie here awake.* For whom are the next twenty minutes more likely to be pleasant—Anne or Janet? Who is under *less* pressure to sleep? What is the impact on the likelihood of returning to sleep of feeling a stronger pressure to sleep? Remember that, as we discussed previously, your reaction to sleeplessness can be more harmful than the sleeplessness itself. Catastrophizing about sleeplessness is not helpful. It makes you more upset in the moment and it keeps you awake longer; in other words, it interferes with sleep.

If worrying about the consequences of poor sleep makes sleep worse, then what is the alternative? One answer is to change what being awake at night means to you. Try this experiment the next time you are awake: Think back to a time when you were awake at the exact same moment you find yourself awake now, when it was actually pleasant. This may be a time when you were out with friends. It may be when your child was born. It may be when you were with someone you love. How would you finish the following sentence? "My best memory of a time when I was awake in the middle of the night is…." If you do not have such a memory, imagine a circumstance in which it would be pleasant to be awake in the night. In either case, spend some time with this pleasant memory or imagined possibility. Close your eyes. Take a deep breath. Allow the memory or image of a pleasant experience of being awake in the middle of the night to unfold, watching it as if it were a movie projected on the insides of your eyelids. Recall or imagine it as vividly as possible. Take in all the scenery. Where were you? Were you with someone? When did this happen? What were you doing? Remember the feeling you had at the time. How do you feel now? Take a deep breath and scan your body. If you notice anxious thoughts about sleeplessness during this exercise, let them be, and return to your pleasant memory. Be open to the pleasant feelings that may arise from focusing on this memory.

Being awake in the middle of the night does not have to be unpleasant. A poor night's sleep does not guarantee feeling horrible the next day. There are times you will have a good night's sleep and feel groggy the next day, and there are times you will sleep horribly yet feel surprisingly well. Remind yourself that although being awake can feel unpleasant, you want to avoid adding to the unpleasantness by becoming highly anxious about it. For more strategies on challenging thoughts that interfere with sleep and accepting wakefulness, read chapters 8 and 9.

Don't Relive the Worst Part of Your Day

Worrying and rumination are often partners in crime in keeping you awake at night. Rumination is like worrying, in that it involves turning information over and over again in your mind. Worrying tends to involve future events; for example, you may worry that you will get fired because of your sleep problems. Rumination tends to focus on past events; for example, you may be thinking about something you said at work and wishing you had said something different. On the surface, figuring out what went wrong and why may seem helpful in preventing similar disasters in the future, but ultimately both worry and rumination lead to feeling worse. Even worse, frequent rumination and worry can become difficult to control.

All the strategies we have discussed so far for dealing with worrying can also be used for dealing with rumination. We now briefly introduce a new strategy that will be elaborated upon in a later chapter—staying focused in the present moment.

If you find yourself reliving the worst part of your day over and over again and you have already left the bedroom but the problem continues, remind yourself that this type of thinking is unhelpful and you need to switch gears and focus on the present moment. Rumination requires attention. To resist rumination, draw your attention away from thoughts of the past by focusing on the here and now. Take a deliberate vacation from your rumination, engage with the here and now, and see how it makes you feel.

How do you do this? First, focus your attention on your breathing. Focus on the sounds and feeling of air moving into your nose, warming your nasal passages, and traveling down into your chest. Now focus on the sounds and feeling of air being moved upward and out of your body. If your attention wanders, do not judge yourself; it is normal for the mind to wander. Instead, gently bring your attention back to your breath. You can build upon this exercise by using the strategies in chapter 10.

Summary

In this chapter, you learned to deal with your worries by setting aside time in the evening to address concerns. If your worries persist at bedtime, take some time to write about your concerns right before bed. Get out of bed if you find yourself worrying or engaging in problem solving in bed and do not return until you have stopped worrying; you will find that, over time, you engage in the worry habit less and less. Remember:

- If your worries persist, generate thoughts and images to distract you from them that are engaging but not too alerting.

- Challenge the idea that being awake at night is a complete catastrophe.

- Counteract rumination and worry by focusing on the present moment.

Chapter 8

Think Like a Good Sleeper

If you have suffered from sleep difficulties for a long time, you may spend more time thinking about sleep than good sleepers do. Preoccupation with sleep makes it difficult for you to quiet your mind, and this contributes to your sleep problems. This chapter will help you identify whether the way you think about sleep could be causing your mental overactivity and sleep problems and will give you the tools you need to manage these unhelpful thoughts.

Signs of Thinking Like a Poor Sleeper

Good sleepers simply do not think very much about sleep. Whereas people who sleep poorly think about their sleep and other life problems when they lie down to sleep, good sleepers report that when they lie down to sleep they think about "nothing in particular." They just go to sleep. In addition to differing from good sleepers in how much they think about sleep, poor sleepers also differ in the way they think about sleep. Are the following thoughts familiar to you?

- *I will have a poor night's sleep.*

- *I cannot manage sleep loss.*

- *If I cannot sleep, I should try harder.*

- *Nothing (short of a miracle drug) could ever help my insomnia.*

- *Monitoring the clock will help me fall asleep more quickly.*

- *My sleep problem is the source of most other problems in my life.*

- *Others should tiptoe around me when I sleep, because I will not be able to fall back asleep if they wake me up.*

- *My tossing in bed at night disturbs my partner (even if my partner has never told me so).*

- *If I do not sleep well on a given night, I will be useless during the day.*

These types of thoughts and beliefs can actually interfere with your ability to sleep. Changing how you think about sleep will help you have fewer sleep-interfering thoughts in bed and pave the way to better sleep.

Take Sleep Loss in Stride

If you woke up in the middle of the night and thought: *Oh no, I can't sleep. I won't be able to fall back asleep; tomorrow will be a tough day,* you would likely feel upset, anxious, or worried. These feelings would make it even harder to fall back asleep. You would probably toss and turn for quite a while.

In contrast, what if you took waking up in stride? For instance, what if you had a matter-of-fact approach and thought: *It seems as if my mind is too active to sleep right now. Trying to force sleep is counterproductive; I am going to go to the couch and watch a sitcom?* Most likely you would be less upset than if you reacted with *Oh no....* Most likely, if you really did take it in stride you would start feeling sleepy while watching one or two sitcom episodes and go back to bed and fall asleep without much tossing and turning.

The way you think about your sleep affects the way you feel, and the way you feel affects your ability to sleep soundly. You may believe that your sleep determines the quality of your life. You may believe that your sleep problems prevent you from enjoying life. Whereas it is true that after a night of poor or insufficient sleep you may not be at your best during the day, the extent to which poor sleep impacts your performance and sense of well-being the next day depends on your reaction to the experience.

If you were to take sleep loss in stride, what would that look like? At night you would remain calm. You might not sleep as much, but you would be resting by calmly engaging in a restful, pleasant experience. You would feel more rested than after an extended struggle with sleep, tossing and turning in bed. During the day you would put thoughts about sleep out of your mind and focus on the day's activities. You might need to alter some behaviors, such as not driving while sleepy, but for the most part you would not change your plans. Moreover, taking sleep in stride means being less distressed, which is always conducive to feeling good during the day and sleeping well at night. The next time you have a night of poor sleep, take it in stride; carry on with your planned activities and see what happens.

Have Realistic Expectations and Beliefs about Sleep

Some poor sleepers think about sleep in an unrealistic or rigid way. There are many common misconceptions about sleep that may lead you to have unrealistic expectations about your sleep. You may not recognize that your expectations are not realistic. Below we discuss how to change a few examples of unrealistic expectations to more realistic ones that could pave the road to better sleep.

I need eight hours or more of sleep. This is an unrealistic belief about sleep because sleep need varies across people, and even for the same person sleep need may not be a constant. For example, when people start a new romantic relationship they tend to sleep considerably less than usual yet still do well during the day—in fact, their life is so exciting that sleep feels like a waste of time. In contrast, when people feel down and depressed they tend to want to sleep for eight hours or more. However, wanting more sleep and needing more sleep are not the same thing. The problem with holding rigidly to the belief that you need eight hours of sleep is that if you sleep for less than eight hours, you may experience anxiety over not having slept "enough."

Within reason, sleep quality is far more important than sleep quantity. You have probably already experienced this truth: think back to a time in which you produced eight hours or more of sleep but did not have optimal mood, energy, or concentration. Or, think back to an occasion on which you had little sleep and were surprised at how well you felt during the day. Read chapter 3 to determine how much time in bed will help you produce the best quality of sleep, and retire the "eight hours of sleep" myth.

I used to have no sleep problems. I should be able to sleep like that again. As we discussed in the previous paragraph, sleep need is not a constant. Moreover, your ability to sleep changes as you age, and it is important that you adjust your expectations accordingly. If you have a middle-aged body, you will be perpetually disappointed if you hold on to the belief that you should have the sleep and energy of a young adult. As you age, the amount of deep sleep you produce decreases and how easily you tire during the day increases. These are normal processes. The consequence of holding on to the unrealistic expectation that you should be able to sleep just the same as when you were younger is that you may become worried that you are not getting enough sleep. You may become anxious at bedtime, which, as we discussed many times in this book, interferes with your ability to sleep. Driven by your worries about sleep, you may try to "fix" your sleep problems in counterproductive ways. In chapters 2 and 3 we discussed a constructive approach to increasing the quality of your sleep, and in chapter 9 we discuss how to increase your energy during the day.

I should fall asleep as soon as my head hits the pillow, and I should stay asleep until morning. Spending up to thirty minutes trying to fall asleep or thirty minutes awake in the middle of the night is considered normal. It is also normal for the brain to briefly wake up many times throughout the night. Most people are unaware of these awakenings or fall quickly back asleep. If your friend tells you that she never wakes up in the middle of the night, she would be more accurate if she said that she is not aware of waking up. People who can sleep at any time, are asleep within minutes, or spend no time awake in bed likely either are very sleep deprived or have an undiagnosed sleep problem such as sleep apnea.

The consequences of having this expectation are similar to those of holding on to other beliefs and expectations we discussed in this section. As minutes pass and you are not asleep yet, you worry that this will be "an insomnia night," and the worry digs you deeper into the hole of having insomnia. Moreover, failure to realize that you have experienced many "normal" nights (i.e., nights in which it takes you thirty minutes or less to fall asleep) convinces you that you are a poor sleeper. Believing that you are and always will be a poor sleeper can become a self-fulfilling prophecy.

Avoid Self-Fulfilling Prophecies

"I feel tense, so I *know* I am never going to be able to sleep." Sound familiar? Hopefully not, because negative predictions are likely to come true. While good sleepers do not think much at all about their sleep, poor sleepers predict that they won't sleep well and then monitor for evidence that their belief was true; that is, they look for proof that they are not sleeping well. They predict that they won't function well during the day and then monitor for evidence of fatigue or difficulty concentrating; often they find such evidence, but simply because they are looking for it. Sleep researchers have never consistently found that a night of poor sleep necessarily means a day of poor functioning, so assuming that it does is neither accurate nor helpful.

Avoid Mental Calculations in the Middle of the Night

If I fall asleep right now, *I will be able to get five hours of sleep...if I fall asleep* now, *I can still get four and a half hours of sleep....* If you become an expert mathematician during the night, constantly calculating how much sleep opportunity you have left, you will be too anxious to ease back into sleep. A team of sleep researchers at the University of California at Berkeley showed that watching the clock makes people think that their sleep is worse than it actually is (Tang,

Schmidt, and Harvey 2007). Avoid the temptation to engage in mental arithmetic at night. Turn your clock around so that you cannot see it.

Avoid Thoughts That Create Performance Anxiety

Performance anxiety occurs in situations in which there is something that you have to do and you worry that you may not be able to do it, or at least do it well. People with insomnia often believe that they must exert effort to sleep. When you are not able to sleep readily, you may become anxious.

Do you believe that when faced with poor sleep you should try harder? Can you sleep only when you don't want to, or when you should not sleep? For example, do you lie awake for most of the night but fall soundly asleep an hour before your alarm is set to go off? (Perhaps you can then sleep after the alarm goes off, knowing that you should really get up to get ready for work.) Or, perhaps you lay your head down after work to rest and find that you sleep for much longer than you intended. Or you doze in the evenings while watching television.

Although some people with sleep problems, no matter how tired, cannot sleep readily under any circumstances, you may find it difficult to resist sleeping under circumstances in which you should not sleep. Then, when you should sleep—that is, at night—you are unable to sleep. Why is it that you can fall asleep when you do not "want" to fall asleep but cannot sleep during conventional hours, when you "want" to sleep?

The answer is this: when there is a demand for sleep, sleep is more difficult to produce. When the pressure to sleep is alleviated, sleep is easier to produce. Nurses often use the following strategy when someone comes to the emergency room in the middle of the night because of an inability to fall asleep. They tell the patient, "The doctor is going to be a while, but please wait up so that you are awake when the doctor comes." This is often successful in facilitating sleep for the patient, as there is now a pressure to stay awake. Similarly, one effective treatment for insomnia, called paradoxical intention, is to ask the person to stay awake all night. In response to this request, the person will often say, "But I do that every night"; however, the attempt to stay awake on purpose is often unsuccessful. The message behind this treatment is that it is easier to sleep when you are not *supposed* to sleep. An effective strategy for this problem is to determine a sleep window as described in chapter 2, and then develop a plan, such as enlisting someone to help make sure that you are awake at all times except during that window. In addition, you can change your thinking about sleep; that is, you can stop *trying* to sleep. If you find yourself awake during the night and it is obvious that you are not going to be able to return to sleep readily, give up the idea that you will try to sleep; instead, get out of bed and don't return until you become sleepy again.

Stop and Question Whether the Thought Is Actually True

You may have noticed a general theme here: that having a thought or belief does not necessarily make it true. Challenging and changing the way you think about your sleep can be as important as challenging or changing your sleep habits. We ask you to stop and question the veracity of your thoughts, because thoughts about sleep can arise automatically. When thoughts are seemingly automatic, you may question whether you can change them at all. You may also believe that because they occur automatically they must somehow be true. Neither of these beliefs is necessarily true. However, if your thoughts about sleep and fatigue are automatic, it will take practice to catch yourself having such thoughts and to actively challenge them. This may be difficult to do, because you may not be aware of your thoughts.

The best way to catch yourself and examine your thoughts may be to notice when your mood worsens—when you become tense or frustrated—and then recall what you were thinking just before your mood changed. Once you identify the thought that is most connected to how you are feeling, ask yourself the following questions:

1. *Is the thought 100 percent true?* (Often thoughts are somewhere between completely true and completely untrue.)

2. *Am I discounting evidence that does not support the thought?*

3. *Am I jumping to conclusions? Am I creating a self-fulfilling prophecy?*

4. *What would I tell someone I loved if he or she was having the same thought?*

5. *Does the thought lead to feeling worse?*

6. *Does the thought lead me to do something that actually interferes with sleep or makes me more apt to feel fatigued?*

Answering these questions and changing your thinking to something more realistic and something that makes you less upset can change your sleep problem. For example, maybe you are used to telling yourself and others, "I don't sleep." Such a thought is inaccurate and anxiety-provoking. If you catch yourself having this thought and you stop to remind yourself that you *do* sleep, albeit less than you would like to, and there are things you can do to sleep even better, this modified thought is more hopeful and adaptive.

Summary

Sometimes the way you think about sleep can make your sleep worse, or at least make it seem worse. This chapter taught you to change the way you think about sleep in several important ways. When you are not overly concerned about sleep loss, refrain from thinking in absolutes such as "I don't sleep," set realistic expectations for your sleep, and avoid thoughts that create anxiety and make it difficult to sleep, you are on your way to thinking like a good sleeper. Try it and enjoy the results! Remember the following tips:

- Take sleep loss in stride.

- One night of poor sleep does not mean the whole week is, or will be, bad.

- Saying "I don't sleep" is inaccurate and increases sleep-related anxiety.

- Sleep is not something that can be produced on demand; believing that you must try to sleep will only make it more difficult to sleep.

- Stop and challenge thoughts that are unhelpful or untrue.

Chapter 9

Focus on the Daytime to Help during the Night

Your sleep problems are not just about your nights; they affect and are affected by your days. Most insomnia sufferers complain less about how they feel at night and more about how they feel during the day. Yet preoccupation with sleep during the day, though understandable, does not solve insomnia; it makes it worse and prolongs the suffering. This chapter gives you tools for modifying your daytime thoughts and actions in order to improve your nights; these include methods to reduce worries, promote acceptance, and challenge unhelpful beliefs about sleep. This chapter also teaches you cognitive skills you can use to help reduce your fatigue and suggests some things you can do during the day to minimize the effects of poor sleep.

Challenge the Myth That Worrying Is Necessary or Helpful

As we discussed in chapter 7, worrying at night can interfere with sleep. Daytime worries can carry over into the night. When facing a worry, ask yourself three questions:

1. *Is this worry about something that has a low probability of actually happening?*

2. *Is this worry about something that is out of my control?*

3. *Is this worry unrealistic or out of proportion?*

If the answer to any of these is yes, then your worrying is not constructive and it is time to challenge this unhelpful habit (this is addressed in the next paragraph and in greater detail in chapter 7). If the answers to all of the above are no, then it may be helpful to turn your attention from worrying to a more action-oriented stance—problem solving. Schedule a private "worry time" (see chapter 7 for a detailed suggestion) to address problems on your mind (but not within an hour or so of your bedtime). You can address the problem by breaking the solution down into manageable steps and identifying the next (immediate) step to take. A common mistake is to ignore the possible intermediate steps; people who make this mistake tend to become overwhelmed and therefore lose confidence in their ability to solve the problem; thinking of the *next* step that you could do today, tomorrow, or sometime this week helps you move toward a solution.

If the answer to any of the above questions is yes, then you are experiencing unproductive worrying. You may engage in this type of worrying because on some level you believe there is some benefit to worrying. Rate the extent to which you believe each of the following statements:

	Do not believe at all	Believe somewhat		Strongly believe
Worrying keeps bad things from happening.	0	1	2	3	4
Better worry now as preparation for when something bad really happens.	0	1	2	3	4
If you don't worry about things it means you don't care.	0	1	2	3	4
Worrying helps you figure out good solutions.	0	1	2	3	4

Each of these beliefs is suspect. Worrying about something that is out of your control will not prevent it from happening. If worrying prevents bad things from happening, then worrying now to minimize your distress later is pointless. Although concern about things that matter to people you care about is one form of expressing your caring, worrying about things that you can do little about ties up energy that you could be investing into other, more productive, ways to express your caring. When you are worried and anxious, you are less available to the people around you. Finally, although worrying can help generate solutions to problems that are solvable, things that are outside of your control or that have a low probability of happening are not solvable problems. Moreover, excessive anxiety can get in the way of putting good solutions into place.

The first step in addressing excessive unproductive worrying, whether about sleep or a myriad of other issues, is to recognize that it is a habit worth changing. Changing this habit requires a commitment to challenging the beliefs that your worrying serves any beneficial purpose and that it is impossible to stop worrying.

Don't Accept Insomnia Myths as Facts

The most common worry of people with insomnia is that they will be unable to cope with the consequences of sleep loss. If you have insomnia, you may be worried that it will lead to some long-term negative health or occupational consequence. After all, sleeping is a basic human function, and it is natural to become anxious when you feel helpless to produce sleep.

147

However, for most people with insomnia these worries are blown out of proportion—that is, they overestimate the likelihood of some future bad consequence. Ask yourself, *What is the evidence that my insomnia will lead to disability or some other negative outcome? What horrible diseases have I contracted so far as a result of my insomnia?* The vast majority of people with clinical insomnia have had untreated or inadequately treated insomnia for years without any major health consequence. If you have heard in the media that sleeping for an average of four hours or less per night is linked to shorter life expectancy, it is important to note that such studies do not assess insomnia; it is therefore not clear whether it is insomnia or other reasons for short sleep duration that underlie this link (Gallicchio and Kalesan 2009). Moreover, the same type of studies also report that sleeping for an average of ten hours or more is also linked to shorter life expectancy. Many people with insomnia do not consistently sleep for only less than four hours. They may experience some very poor nights with little sleep, but they usually also experience some nights with more sleep, and their average sleep time is usually more than four hours.

To help you gain some perspective on worries that your insomnia will have catastrophic consequences, consider what advice you would give to a friend or family member in the same position. Would you advise your friend or family member to worry about it? Would you say, "Yes, you're probably right, you are heading for an early grave..."? Probably not. Most likely you understand that such a statement would only increase your friend or family member's worry and make sleep even more difficult. You would probably recognize that your friend or family member's worry was excessive. Since insomnia is a common problem, you probably know quite a few people with insomnia. Do you see disproportionate rates of illness and disability and death among your friends and family members who have trouble sleeping? Would you believe that your friend with insomnia was going to contract a disease or meet an early death just because of her sleep problems? Probably not. These realizations should make it easier for you to respond to friends and family members who anticipate catastrophic consequences of poor sleep in a calm and supportive manner, helping them put things in perspective. Can you consider a similar approach to your own beliefs?

The previous hypothetical exercise highlights two points: first, beliefs about catastrophic outcomes of poor sleep are not very accurate; second, they are not very useful. Worrying makes it more likely that you will be too anxious to sleep well. Moreover, worrying increases muscle tension that leads to physical fatigue, and it uses valuable mental resources, resulting in mental fatigue. Over time, worrying about the consequences of poor sleep may become the main cause of prolonged chronic insomnia. This is an important point that is surprising to most people; that is, irrespective of what initially caused your sleep problems, worrying about sleep may have become the number one factor sustaining your current sleep problems. It is therefore important that you find ways to reduce your worries about sleep. This is not an easy task. We hope that our discussion below will be helpful in this regard.

Challenge Your Beliefs by Doing the Opposite

Sometimes people with sleep problems act in ways that unintentionally strengthen unhelpful beliefs about their sleep. For example, if you believe that you have a limited ability to cope with the daytime consequences of poor sleep and you tend to cancel plans or avoid activities after a poor night's sleep, then you are reaffirming the idea that you are unable to cope with the sleep loss. If you continue to respond to poor sleep with this strategy, your schedule will become more irregular, you may become less active, and you may even be prone to spending more time in bed; all of these behaviors have been found to prolong the very sleep problems you are trying to solve.

An alternative, and potentially better, approach is to challenge your belief in your limited ability to cope with the daytime consequences of poor sleep by carrying out your regular activities despite the fact that you have not slept well. This may require you to change your mind-set and to use new coping strategies. For example, be sure to eat well and regularly, keep hydrated, plan to take breaks when doing boring or monotonous activities (as we discuss later in this chapter), and be sure to inject some fun into your day as well. Good sleepers take bad nights in stride and proceed with their regularly scheduled activities. If you are unable to follow this advice because you strongly believe that you have a fixed and low amount of energy from which to draw upon during the day, test this belief by spending a week conserving your energy all day, every day. Rest as much as you can and track your hourly energy levels, your mood, and the quality of your sleep. Then spend a week expending your energy. Do the things that you would do if you had slept well even if you feel as if your energy reserve is low. Track your energy levels, your sleep, and your mood for this week too. You will likely be surprised at what you learn.

Fatigue—Don't Let It Stop You!

Fatigue—feeling mentally, physically, or emotionally tired—is the number one complaint of people with sleep problems. Under normal conditions, resting or taking a nap helps with fatigue; but when difficulty sleeping becomes chronic, resting rarely helps improve energy levels and, as we discussed in the previous paragraph, it may increase the likelihood that your sleep and fatigue problems will continue or worsen.

If you feel mentally fatigued after a poor night's sleep, you may doubt that you will be able to perform your everyday duties adequately. You may worry that you will make a mistake at work that will cause you to look bad or even to lose your job. If you are responsible for looking after young children, you may worry about whether you will be able to pay close enough attention to keep them safe.

Luckily, we know that although greater effort than usual is required, people with sleep problems continue to perform routine mental tasks normally. Although you may not feel very sharp after a night of poor sleep, you are unlikely to be impaired when performing routine activities. If you are concerned about memory impairment, you may want to use external aids to memory, such as to-do lists, leaving sticky notes in prominent places to remind you to do something, or asking someone to remind you. Sticking to your routines, using such aids when needed, is preferable to calling in sick to work or otherwise avoiding your responsibilities. Remember that, as we discussed in the previous section, avoiding or canceling activities can reinforce the idea that you are incapable of coping with sleep loss, a belief that will increase your anxiety about your sleep problems.

Feeling physically fatigued can make it difficult to get out of bed in the morning, stay out of bed in the evening, exercise or perform normal physical activities, and avoid trying to nap. Whereas normally you would rest to manage fatigue, in the context of sleep problems resting rarely makes you feel better; it may even make you feel more fatigued. This is because inactivity breeds more inactivity. An object at rest tends to stay at rest. Or more succinctly, an object on the couch tends to stay on the couch. Inactivity can have negative effects on sleep and can worsen fatigue. Keep to your normal routine if you can, and address the common causes of fatigue listed later in this chapter.

Some people who sleep poorly tend to assume that when they do not feel well during the day or they perform poorly it must be due to poor sleep, ignoring other possible causes. Don't make lack of sleep a scapegoat. Have you not, after all, had okay days after a poor night's sleep? Conversely, have you never felt bad or performed poorly after a good night's sleep? Does having a really good night's sleep always prevent feeling bad during the day? The fact is that daytime problems and sleep are not as perfectly related as you might think. Importantly, there are negative consequences to blaming poor mood, fatigue, and concentration problems exclusively on sleep. Here are some tips to help you avoid this trap.

Avoid Appraising Your Sleep within an Hour of Waking Up

During the first thirty to sixty minutes after waking up, you may be experiencing what is called sleep inertia or sleep drunkenness. Feeling groggy and tired upon waking may have nothing to do with the amount or quality of your sleep. You may have woken up from a deep stage of sleep. You may have awoken from a dream. Your body clock type may also contribute to sleep inertia. In comparison to a morning person (an "early bird"), who tends to feel wide awake and alert upon awakening, a night person (a "night owl") takes a long time to feel optimally alert. All of the above, and more, are possible explanations for feeling poor upon waking up in the morning. It would therefore be a mistake to conclude that feeling bad in the morning means that your sleep was of poor quality or insufficient.

Imagine that two men, Dan and Stan, have both been awakened by an alarm from a deep stage of sleep. Dan thinks: *Whew, I'm sleepy; I must have been in a deep sleep. I'd better get into the shower and shake this feeling off.* Stan thinks: *Whew, I'm sleepy; I must have had another bad night. I'd better stay in bed and try to get more sleep.* Which of these reactions would likely lead to feeling worse during the day? Who will have greater sleep anxiety—Dan or Stan? Which of the two is more likely to have sleep problems in the future?

Address the Common Causes of Fatigue

There are many reasons for feeling tired other than insufficient or poor-quality sleep. The good news is that most of these factors are well within your control and may be simple to fix. Understand the following common causes of fatigue and address them.

The "boomerang" effect of caffeine. You may rely on caffeinated beverages like energy drinks, pop, tea, or coffee to make you feel more alert when you feel fatigued. These beverages may initially help you feel an energy boost. However, you may later experience a drop in energy, or a caffeine "crash." Worse is the fact that the crash may be (mis)interpreted as due to your sleep problems, rather than the metabolism of the caffeine, which is entirely unrelated to sleep. In other words, you may have felt tired mid-morning and had a latte to keep you going, then several hours later felt tired again and thought, "I can't take how my problems sleeping make me feel tired all the time." This and other inaccurate attributions increase your anxiety about sleep, making it difficult for you to approach sleep in a casual, effortless way (like a good sleeper; see chapter 8). Moreover, if later in the day you continue consuming caffeine, it might directly interfere with your ability to fall asleep, depending on how close it is to your bedtime and how sensitive you are to the alerting effects of caffeine. Consider cutting back or eliminating your caffeine intake.

The "post-lunch dip." Have you ever noticed a dip in your energy, alertness, or mood in the early part of the afternoon? Most people blame this phenomenon on a big lunch. However, you should know that your level of alertness is controlled in part by your body clock. Your body temperature naturally rises and falls over a twenty-four-hour course, and you are most sleepy when your temperature is falling. The most prominent dip in temperature occurs at night, but there is one brief occasion during the day when most people's body temperature falls slightly, usually sometime between noon and three. This dip in energy levels is temporary. Now consider two ways of reacting to this dip:

1. Believing that this midday energy dip means that your fatigue is increasing and this is a sign that you did not sleep well or for long enough

2. Believing that it is a brief, temporary natural dip that is unrelated to your sleep problems

Which of these two reactions will produce more anxiety about sleep? Which is more likely to result in helpful, adaptive behaviors? Given the earlier discussion about caffeine, which of these two reactions is going to lead people to re-caffeinate after lunch? If you can weather the "post-lunch dip" without caffeine, you will see your energy levels naturally rise again and you will be more likely to get good sleep later.

Inactivity. What do you feel like doing when you are tired? Probably not much at all. When you are tired, it makes sense to rest; however, when you have chronic sleep problems, this natural inclination to rest leads to greater levels of fatigue. In physics, as we noted above, an object at rest tends to stay at rest, because of inertia. The same is true of people who stay at rest. Why? Because inactivity breeds more fatigue, until it is difficult to do anything.

When you engage in physical activity, your metabolism speeds up and your body releases endorphins, both of which give you more energy. Exercise has health and sleep benefits, but overactivity and physical exertion can produce fatigue, so try to find a balance. Movement and regular light physical activity is a good start to reduce fatigue and improve sleep.

Poor nutrition or irregular meals. You need appropriate nutrients from foods in order to maintain energy in your body. Certain weight-loss diets, such as those low in carbohydrates, can deprive your body of vital nutrients and fuel that you need to get through the day.

Eat too little and your blood sugar will fall; eat too much and your blood sugar will spike. A diet high in sugar will negatively impact your blood sugar levels and result in high levels of fatigue and mental cloudiness. Eating regular, well-portioned meals will manage fatigue related to blood sugar levels.

Irregular bowel movements are linked with many health problems and symptoms like fatigue. When you are constipated, toxins in your body are not being eliminated properly. The toxins can thus build up and demand more of your body's energy to process and store. Constipation often can be alleviated with changes in diet. Talk about recurring constipation with your health care provider.

Anemia. The body needs iron to function properly. If your blood iron levels are low (a condition called anemia), your heart and other vital organs may be receiving less oxygen than they should, which can drain your energy and cause mild to severe fatigue. If you have ulcers, heavy menstrual flow, or hemorrhoids, or if you are taking NSAIDS (nonsteroidal anti-inflammatory drugs) such as ibuprofen, you may be at increased risk of anemia. Your physician can check for anemia with a simple blood test. You can also ask your physician to check for deficiencies of vitamins such as B_{12}. Vitamin B_{12} levels typically decline with age, particularly for men, and low B_{12} can be associated with high levels of fatigue. If you have had anemia in the past, it is important to note that anemia can and in fact often does return.

Dehydration. Your body is composed mostly of water, and you need to keep it replenished. You may or may not need eight glasses every day, but the fact is that people tend to not drink enough water. If your water intake is too low, you can become dehydrated, which affects your energy levels. Preventing dehydration, which is very important for your general health, is thus also an effective fatigue management strategy. Note that caffeinated beverages have a diuretic (dehydrating) effect, so caffeine drinkers need even more water than others to compensate.

Boredom. Boredom is often underestimated as a source of fatigue. If you don't believe that engaging in mundane activities without adequate breaks can be fatiguing, think of how it feels to stare at a computer screen for hours on end. There is nothing physically taxing about using a computer, and you are resting in a chair while doing it, so why does it make you feel so tired? The reason is because levels of sustained activity can cause muscle soreness and eye strain and lead to mental and physical fatigue. Take frequent breaks from mundane activities, particularly those involving your eyes.

Treatable mood problems. Certainly if you have depression, but even if you don't, there is a close relationship between low mood and low energy. When you feel down, you are more likely to feel fatigued. There is also a vicious circle wherein the lower your mood, the more tired you feel, and the less you feel like doing anything; the less you do, the more likely you are to feel tired. Combat temporary low mood by distracting yourself and doing things that make you feel more positive. If your mood is more pervasive, you may be experiencing depression and should seek help. Depression is treatable.

Inadequately treated or managed pain. Dealing with pain uses physical and emotional energy, which can cause you to feel fatigued. In addition, some conditions that cause pain may also cause fatigue.

Seek treatment for pain. Pain is manageable through a variety of approaches. This may include pain medications; there are a variety of non-narcotic medications available if you do not wish to take potentially addictive medications. Additionally there are proven psychotherapeutic approaches, including cognitive behavioral therapy for pain, that teach physical, mental, and behavioral techniques for addressing pain.

Talk to your health care provider about safe ways for you to continue to be active despite pain; it will help you manage fatigue as well as secondary pain (the pain that comes from consequences of inadequate activity, such as muscle shortening or deconditioning).

Anxiety and stress. There can be a cycle in which you have sleep problems that make you anxious or create stress and the resultant anxiety or stress worsens and maintains your sleep problems. The same can be said of anxiety about fatigue. The more anxious you are about what your fatigue means for your future functioning, the greater your levels of fatigue will be.

Even if you are not explicitly anxious or stressed about your sleep problems, you may be someone who generally experiences high levels of stress and anxiety. People who are overly anxious or stressed keep their bodies in overdrive. The body often uses adrenaline to deal with anxiety and stresses, which, over time, causes fatigue to set in. The fatigue can also relate to chronic muscle tension. Attributing fatigue to sleep problems rather than anxiety may keep you from properly addressing an anxiety or stress-related problem. Follow the guidelines in chapter 6 to establish a relaxation practice and you will no doubt notice a reduction in your fatigue levels.

Immune system or allergic response. Fatigue can be brought on by bacterial or viral infections such as colds and flus, autoimmune reactions, and food aller-gies. Your body uses a lot of energy to fight infection and deal with what it identifies as unwanted foreign substances, thus leaving you feeling fatigued. It is important not to assume that fatigue is related to poor sleep when it could relate to a treatable infection or an allergy.

Hormone-related problems. In most cases, fatigue is a benign symptom, but it is also a fairly nonspecific symptom of many more troublesome disorders. Whenever you are faced with chronic fatigue, tell your doctor. Ask your doctor to check for some common hormonal imbalance disorders such as hypothyroid-ism, which is characterized by an underactive thyroid. Hypothyroidism can cause fatigue and is relatively easily treated with medication.

Summary

This chapter discussed how taking a second look at your beliefs that worrying is helpful and that having had a sleepless night handicaps you during the day can help you get better sleep in the future. It also provided a wake-up call that maybe your problems are about more than just sleep (or lack thereof). When you take steps to address other possible causes of fatigue and try to stay active and have a normal day in spite of insomnia, you will benefit. Don't forget:

- Question your worries.

- Look for all the other common reasons for fatigue, rather than exclusively blaming sleep for how you feel during the day.

- It is normal to sometimes feel sleepy for up to an hour after waking up.

- Drink plenty of water; eat regular, well-balanced meals; and get regular physicals to check for fatigue-related problems such as vitamin deficiencies or hypothyroidism.

- Avoid rest or inactivity as a response to fatigue resulting from insomnia.

- Ward off fatigue that is the product of boredom and eye strain by taking breaks from monotonous activities.

Chapter 10

Accept and Be Willing: What You Resist Persists

So far we have given you tools to help you work with, rather than against, your body's natural sleep system. We have given you tools to manage unwanted thoughts and worrying, anxiety, and other thoughts that worsen your sleep problems and/or fatigue. Some of these tools require practice and consistency before their full effect is felt. If you find it difficult to use one or more of these effective tools consistently, it may be because thoughts and feelings about your sleep problems get in the way. If this is the case, you may find this chapter particularly helpful. This final chapter discusses the important role of acceptance and willingness in helping you quiet your mind.

The Finger-Trap

You are probably no stranger to lying awake frustrated at not being able to sleep. When this happens, does your mind go around and around thinking about how you can get rid of your sleep problems or wondering why they persist? Do you notice things that interfere with your sleep, such as nervousness in your stomach, thoughts that won't stop, bothersome noises, and pain in your body? Perhaps you do not think of sleep at all. You may be thinking about your day, tomorrow's activities, or that you do not like lying awake.

Sleep problems can be frustrating and even upsetting. However, the greater your frustration and distress, the more difficult it is to sleep. So, should you try to *pretend* that you are not upset by your sleep problems? Not exactly.

Have you ever had your fingers caught in a Chinese finger-trap? The way a Chinese finger-trap works is this: You place your index fingers in each end of a soft woven tube and then your task is to get your fingers out. As you try to pull your fingers out, you notice that your fingers are gripped more tightly—you are trapped. The harder you pull your fingers, the tighter the tube becomes, making it impossible to escape. Brute force only makes the situation worse.

The solution to the finger-trap is a paradox. When you resist the urge to fight the trap and instead relax into it by pushing your fingers farther into the tube, you create more space and can release your fingers. When you choose to no longer struggle, trusting that it will be okay, the trap opens and you are free.

Think about difficulty falling asleep. The harder you try to sleep, the more elusive sleep becomes. As is the case for a Chinese finger-trap, the solution is to change tactics; rather than trying harder, relax into it. We are not talking about giving up. We are saying that a willingness to experience wakefulness and fatigue, rather than resisting them, may be necessary in order to get out of the sleeplessness trap.

Learn How to Accept

Jason Ong, PhD, is director of the Behavioral Sleep Medicine Program at Rush University Medical Center in Chicago. In his innovative mindfulness-based treatment for insomnia, he uses the poem "The Guest House" by Rumi to teach acceptance. "The Guest House," which describes people as houses, suggests that emotion—whether joy, tension, frustration, or anxiety—is a visitor to be welcomed into your house. Welcoming unpleasant emotions and experiences such as wakefulness in the middle of the night, an overactive mind, frustration, fatigue, or tension may at first seem an unusual suggestion. However, the fact is that these unwanted guests are already at your doorstep. You may want them to leave, but you have little control over whether they will actually leave. Attempting to control that which you have little control over allows unwanted thoughts and feelings to dominate your house. Perhaps you can consider an alternative approach, much like the solution to the Chinese finger-trap. Invite bothersome thoughts or feelings, such as worry, frustration, anxiety, anger, sadness, or fatigue, into your house. This will put you in a calmer state of mind, opening the door to the guest you really want: sleep.

Be Open to Being Awake

"The Guest House" reminds us that being invested in making something *not* happen makes it more likely to happen. Trying to make something not happen takes up an enormous amount of energy and focus. What if you were open to being awake during the night? If you were open to the experience, you wouldn't be as upset when it happened. In fact it is likely that you would still be calm enough to soon fall asleep.

Understand that being open to a situation is not the same as being happy about it—the suggestion is to be at peace with the way things are. Understand and accept that there is little you can do, and choose not to devote any more energy to resistance.

There is nothing inherently disastrous about being awake at night. Think of a time when being awake during the night was enjoyable. Think of one of your first sleepovers or when you spent the night with someone you love. In these instances it was enjoyable to stay up at night. When you cannot sleep, challenge the part of your experience that says, "This is horrible." Instead, choose to engage in something enjoyable and peaceful outside the bed (see chapter 4 for suggestions) and you will have a different experience.

Be Open to Feeling Tired during the Day

After a night of poor sleep, you may feel tired. You may feel unmotivated and have trouble concentrating. You may think, *I am never going to be able to make it through today*, leading you to call in sick to work, cancel or avoid certain activities, attempt to sleep in, or take a long daytime nap.

In the same way that you can choose to accept being awake during the night, rather than staying stuck in a struggle against the experience, you can choose to accept feelings of tiredness during the day, rather than giving in to these feelings and reducing your activity levels.

If you choose to accept feelings of tiredness during the day, you can turn your attention to ways to cope with fatigue. What if, in the spirit of "The Guest House," you were to say to yourself: *Okay, so tiredness is here; that's fine. Tiredness is an unwelcome guest, but it is not going to stop me from doing what I normally do. I'll control what I can. I will take frequent breaks from my work to manage eye fatigue/strain and boredom; I will get fresh air to provide mini-bursts of energy; I will drink lots of water to avoid caffeine and the crash that inevitably follows; I will accept that today may or may not be a difficult day because of the way I am feeling. It's okay.* Try to adopt an accepting stance toward fatigue this week and notice the transformation in your experience.

Live in the Moment: The Time Is Now

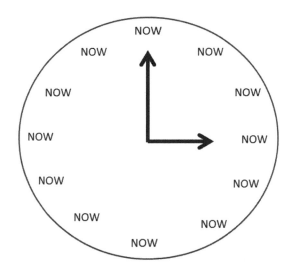

When you worry, you focus on the future: you fear that something bad will happen and you will be ill-equipped to deal with it. If you are concerned that you will not sleep tonight, that tomorrow will be a bad night because of how poorly you slept, or that you will never recover from your sleep problems, you are focusing on a future that may or may not happen. A considerable amount of misery is attached to thinking about the future rather than your present reality. There is a simple solution to this unhelpful habit.

The solution is found in the present moment. You cannot know what will happen in the future, but the present moment is certain. There are no disasters in the room at the moment—only imagined ones in the future. Take a moment right now, at this moment, and notice what is around you. What do you notice about your surroundings? What do you hear? What do you smell? How does the temperature feel on your skin? If you are sitting, tune in to the places where your body comes in contact with the chair. If you are standing, focus on your feet touching the ground. What do you notice? Listen to your breathing. Feel the air move into your nose or mouth and down into your chest. Awaken your awareness to the present moment. The current moment is peaceful, and the current moment is more helpful for sleep than either the past or the future. Being mindful of the moment will help you accept what the current moment brings.

Practice Mindfulness by Creating Mindful Moments

Becoming more presently aware in the moment takes practice. One of the pitfalls to watch out for as you develop this skill is impatience. As you try to increase your awareness and be in the moment, your attention may stray. A common reaction to realizing that your attention has strayed is to become frustrated and become tempted to give up. Yet, the moment you realize that your attention has strayed is a moment of increased awareness of the present; this is part of the process and an opportunity for you to calmly redirect your attention to the present moment. Be patient; mindfulness takes time to develop. Remember Jon Kabat-Zinn's parachute analogy from chapter 6, and think of taking the time to cultivate this skill as weaving your parachute.

Look for opportunities to increase your awareness for brief periods throughout your day. Instead of letting your mind wander as you stroke your pet, do the dishes, or take a walk, be mindful of the sights, sounds, smells, and feelings in the present moment as you do these things. Stroke your pet mindfully; do the dishes mindfully; go for a walk mindfully. These exercises will train your mind to focus less on past mistakes that cannot be undone and future disasters that may never come and to focus more on what is happening right now. You can use any activity you like to help you practice mindfulness. Activities that involve all of your senses tend to work best. Below are two examples of turning mundane experiences into exercises in mindfulness: eating mindfully and bathing mindfully. Developing this new habit of mind could eventually help you tame your active mind at night.

Eat a Meal Mindfully

Eating is an activity that can and often does becomes automatic. Automatic eating can diminish your enjoyment of food and can also promote overeating, if physiological cues that you are getting full or were not really hungry to begin with are ignored. Eating a meal mindfully, on the other hand, can awaken your senses and help you pay closer attention to other experiences throughout the day. It can be a break from the tension and stress of your day. Mindful eating is a way to connect with your body and take in the current moment. There are no emergencies during a meal—just eating.

For this exercise, pick a time when you can eat alone, without being disturbed. Prepare yourself a meal and sit down comfortably to eat, but before you pick up a utensil or lift the food to your lips, close your eyes. Take a deep breath and notice the sensation of the air moving over your lips or nostrils and traveling down into your chest. Maybe the breath moves even deeper, down into your belly. Now focus your attention on the breath leaving your body. Repeat this two or more times. If you become distracted, gently return your attention to your breath. Now, look down at what you are about to eat. Notice how it looks: the colors, the shapes, the textures. What will you eat first? Take your time deciding, but when you do, focus your attention and explore the item with your eyes. What do you notice? Then engage your sense of smell. Does what you are about to eat have an enticing aroma? Focus your attention on your nose and how it draws air up into the nasal passages. Notice whether you are holding a fork or a spoon. Focus on the feeling of the points of contact of the utensil with your skin. Are you gripping it tightly, loosely, or somewhere in between? Move toward the food and pick it up with your fork or spoon. Take your time. Bring the food to your mouth and pause. What do you notice now about the food that you didn't when it was on your plate—what do you see; what do you smell? Imagine what the food will taste like. Put the food into your mouth, but don't chew yet. Take time to notice how it feels on your tongue. Now slowly and deliberately start chewing, paying attention to the movement of your jaws and mouth. Chew slowly at least twenty times. What do you notice about the movement of your mouth? What do you notice about the taste of the food? What do you notice about swallowing? Take your time and repeat these steps for your entire meal.

Take a Bath Mindfully

Taking a mindful bath is a popular way to practice mindfulness because it serves an additional purpose: getting clean. Although most people find taking a bath relaxing, relaxation is not the goal of mindfulness exercises. The purpose of mindful bathing and other mindfulness exercises is becoming mindful—indeed, because becoming mindful takes practice, these exercises may not be relaxing at all.

When you have filled the tub with water and settled comfortably in, start your mindful bath by focusing your attention on your breathing. Because of the acoustics in your bathroom, your breathing may sound different from the way it normally does. Or perhaps your ears are submerged, so your hearing experience is completely different than usual. Whatever the case, focus your attention on your breath for several moments. Then move gently in the tub and notice the sounds that result. Do you hear a drip? Do you hear a tiny bit of water escaping down the drain? What else do you notice? What do you notice about the temperature of the water? What do you notice about the skin temperature of parts of your body that are sticking out of the water? Now slowly begin to wash yourself, turning your attention to how each of the steps in bathing feels. Pay attention to the way it feels to lather soap on your body, the smells of the soap mixing with your natural body odors, and how the lather looks. Watch the water bead off your body as you wash away the soap. Take your time and notice each part of this experience.

Observe Your Thoughts

Perhaps you are reading this book because you have an overactive mind in general. Try as you will to shut it off, sometimes the thoughts keep coming, and their presence becomes more and more frustrating.

You feel trapped by your thoughts and you want to escape. On these occasions it is as if your thoughts are a rushing current, pulling you downriver as you struggle to reach the bank. What if, instead, you could sit on the riverbank and observe your thoughts without getting caught up in them?

Try this exercise. When a thought comes to mind, simply notice it and imagine the words of the thought being written on a leaf. Imagine placing the leaf on a stream and watching it float away until it disappears around a bend. Here comes another thought (leaf). Notice it. Notice the words on the leaf as it floats away. If you notice any negative emotion, accept that it is there; notice it without judgment; gently turn your attention to observing your thoughts once more. Do this as often as necessary; that is, whenever you notice yourself distracted, refocus your attention. If critical thoughts about how this exercise is unfolding arise, put those on leaves too and set them adrift.

You can choose other images similar to the idea of a leaves on a stream. For example, you can put your thoughts on clouds that you watch drift away, on signs in a parade that you watch march past, or on bubbles that you watch float upward.

Create Moments of Zen in Chaos

A common myth about meditation is that you need to have a quiet mind in order to be successful. On the contrary, meditation is about acceptance. In meditation, a quiet mind has no greater value than a noisy mind—both are met with acceptance and with a curious, observing spirit. The concepts of "success" and "failure" are foreign to mindfulness. Mindfulness is about watching your thoughts, however noisy they are and regardless of how upsetting they may be.

The practice of observing your thoughts can, over time, decrease the likelihood that you will become caught up in your thoughts. Think of those scenes in cartoons and movies in which a central character is surrounded by chaos—when suddenly everything slows down. In this moment of slow motion, the central character is able to create some stillness to take a break and gather himself or herself. Wouldn't it be nice to do this in real life? Mindfulness offers you such a break.

"Zen" refers to a meditative state that you can achieve for brief periods throughout your day. When things are stressful and chaotic, take a moment to sit down. Go somewhere you can be alone for a moment to shut your eyes and breathe (maybe the bathroom). Pay attention to your breath for a minute. Creating a breathing space can give you the break you need to compose yourself, re-center, and reconnect with your strength and coping skills.

You can do this any time you want; take a few minutes away from work or other stressful tasks to practice mindfulness, and observe how you feel afterward. Mindfulness is a practice wherein you become more awake and more aware—this can have positive effects on your levels of alertness. Take short mindfulness breaks throughout your day, and observe the difference in your mental alertness.

Summary

This chapter explained how acceptance can help you be more at peace with the way things are. If you can accept, for example, that you are having difficulty falling asleep and remember that being awake at night is not always a bad thing, you will likely fall asleep sooner than if you resisted the idea of being awake in a spirit of frustration. Likewise, if you accept that you may feel tired during the day, fatigue is no longer your enemy.

Mindfulness helps you change the experience of worry and rumination by increasing your focus on the present moment. It takes practice, but once you develop a habit of mindfulness, you will be more accepting of your sleep problems and they will cease to loom so large in your mind. Remember the following tips:

- Be open to being awake at night.

- Be open to being tired during the day.

- Live in the moment.

- Create mindful moments during your day.